How can you avoid and reverse free radical damage in your own body?

THIS BOOK PROVIDES THE ANSWERS:
Just as oxidation turns apples brown, a similar process in your own body triggers reactions that lead to disease and the symptoms of aging. The agents that act as triggers can be pollutants, low-level radiation, chemical contaminants, stress—all the harmful by-products of modern life. But now there's a comprehensive guide, the first of its kind, to advise you on the preventative and protective measures you need. *Good Health in a Toxic World* reveals how the appropriate diet, vitamin supplements, mental attitude, exercise, antioxidants, pollution avoidance, and exposure to full-spectrum light empower you—in the face of environmental toxicity—to take charge of and preserve your health.

"Fascinating reading, and very well researched. This is the first book to offer clear, reliable guidance to help us avoid the dangers of excess free radicals. An easy-to-follow and practical guide to healthy living. A 'must read.'"
—Nathaniel Altman, author of *Sacred Trees*

"A comprehensive guide to developing optimal health and specifically how to counteract health-depleting free radicals. Well documented, and offers valuable resources and terrific recipes."
—Jon Naar, author of *This Land Is Your Land*

"I have never read a book that has more to say about staying young and healthy. And says it so clearly and concisely. A refresher for the mind and body."
—Jess Stearn, author of *The Power of Alpha Thinking*

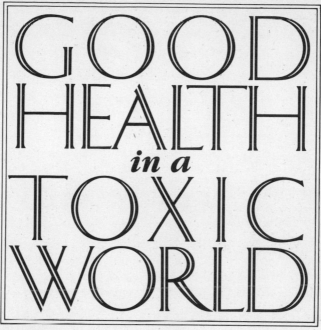

GOOD HEALTH *in a* TOXIC WORLD

The Complete Guide to Fighting Free Radicals

SARA SHANNON

WARNER BOOKS

A Time Warner Company

Copyright © 1994 by Sara Shannon
All rights reserved.

Warner Books, Inc., 1271 Avenue of the Americas, New York, NY 10020

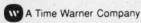 A Time Warner Company

Printed in the United States of America
First Printing: October 1994
10 9 8 7 6 5 4 3 2 1

Library of Congress Cataloging-in-Publication Data
Shannon, Sara.
    Good health in a toxic world : the complete guide to fighting free radicals / Sara Shannon.
        p.   cm.
    Includes bibliographical references.
    ISBN 0-446-67005-7
    1. Free radicals (Chemistry)—Pathophysiology.   2. Active oxygen in the body.   3. Antioxidants—Health aspects.   4. Medicine, Preventive.   I. Title.
RB170.S53   1994
616.07—dc20   94-21777
                                                                      CIP

Book design by H. Roberts

Cover design by Christine Van Bree

This book is dedicated to Mother Nature, with thanks for the abundance she lays at our feet in hopes that we use it with the reverence it deserves.

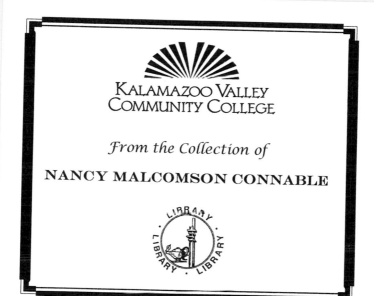

CONTENTS

FOREWORD

by Dan Roehm

*I*n her first book, *Diet for the Atomic Age*, Sara Shannon, a responsible mother and pioneer nutritionist, tells us how when in 1979 she first got news of the disastrous accident at Three Mile Island nuclear plant in Pennsylvania, "My instinct spoke to me," and she made plans to evacuate New York City, some 170 miles away, with her grade school son despite the pooh-poohs of officialdom from President Carter (an Annapolis–trained nuclear engineer) on down. Yet Shannon was right and the experts were wrong. Although she doesn't say so, the same above operant phrase "My instinct spoke to me" next caused Shannon to listen and just "know" there had to be foods that confer upon us protection from radioactivity. Official opinion said no to this too, but again she was proven right by further research. When she scratched beneath the surface, she learned that Nature was chock-full of foods that helped the body do the seemingly impossible in ridding itself of radioactive materials—e.g., sodium alginate from kelp separated strontium-90 in the intestines from the nearly similar calcium atom. She found that various plant fibers and substances such as phytates were also reported effective in this *if* you knew where to look buried in the scattered scientific literature. Shannon knew where to look, and she knew how to bring it together in this book.

In the present book, *Good Health in a Toxic World*, Shannon comes before us to tell that although free radical destructiveness is seen most pristinely in radiation damage, it stalks us every day of our lives and still would even if we were not daily exposed to significant radiation—a utopian state impossible in this country since 1946—and is the direct mediator of all our degenerative diseases and "normal aging process." Despite the degree of *accelerated* bodily dissolution observable in our society, society, in the main, still does not make the connection between good nutrition, a healthy lifestyle, and excellent health.

Most readers of this book are likely to be familiar with the term "free radicals" and their counteracting "antioxidants" and yet they may feel somehow left out from a serviceable understanding of what it is all about. Why do we have free radicals in the first place? Why does our friend, oxygen, have to exist in a vicious species such as "singlet oxygen" or "hydroxyl free radicals," which requires antioxidants guarding against it?

The answer is that without the high energy that controlled free radicals can provide our bodies we would lose our present high level of bodily performance: among other things we would move about with muscles propelling us slower than snails and our white blood cells could not zap invading bacteria and viruses (who themselves have their own "free rads" to zap us)—our quality of life would be unbearably sickly, slow, and dull.

What is happening on planet Earth is that people are far too tired and more listless than they should be, their immune systems are so depressed they cannot dispatch invading cells (including cancer) as their ancestors once could and many of our babies soon slip into a state of chronic fatigue and illness that prevent them from experiencing the joy of being young, fresh, and vibratingly alive because they can no longer maintain themselves in this blessed state which is their birthright. To top it off, our highly trained MDs offer totally malapropos measures which can do virtually nothing to help you with this. Drugs are not the answer to free radicals. The right lifestyle is. There is great promise in the informative books now appearing, of which this is one of the best. It is unique in explaining what free radicals are, what causes them, and how you can counteract them. It shows you on almost every page how inept the orthodox medical profession is in pushing antibiotics and other drugs that are always two-edged swords and often totally irrelevant to the problems of a population that is insidiously chronically ill and has long forgotten what wellness is, if, indeed, they have ever experienced it. Down, down, down goes the average state of health in our citizenry who have been led to believe our medical care is good and that our increase in longevity is due to the miracles of modern medicine. It isn't. Our life expectancy *after we reach fifty* has increased little since mid-century when the supposed blessings of antibiotics, chemotherapy, and bypass surgery have kicked in. After fifty is when the degenerative diseases get into full swing, though there are plenty of people in their early forties now who are much further along in their "normal aging process" than the calendar tells them.

No, our bumper crop of senior citizens today is largely due to the conquering of various epidemic diseases of childhood, which were mainly brought under control in the first quarter of this century by engineering means, *not* medical ones: better housing, transportation, sewage disposal, etc.

Having practiced as an internist/cardiologist for nearly half a century (with heavy but belated emphasis on nutrition during the last decade of this time), I have also seen the nearly total disappearance in our population of people in "radiant good health" (these I saw mostly in my childhood and they were usually just off the farm or still on it).

Yet I am happy to report that in my practice there was *one* "sub-set" (a biostatistician's term) of the population that was old, but who were pickers-up of their feet as they walked, alert, strong, largely pain free, sexy, who could be termed "spry" (although not by me, they were young enough in body and spirit so they could cuff you if you dared call them that) and those are the ones who invariably have been "on vitamins" and "natural foods," i.e., into preventive nutrition for at least a decade. They looked (and were, biologically, which is all that concerns us here) ten to fifteen years younger than their year of birth indicated. Did they ever enjoy fooling the doctor on this—someone whom they rarely needed to see and often didn't much like. They were very well read, by the way.

In short, they were playing a great game called "free radical control" long before science discovered free radicals. They did this, I am convinced, because like Sara Shannon they experienced something like "My instinct spoke to me."

But one small sub-set is not enough—not everyone has these inner promptings, or, if they do, they don't listen. We always will need such people as Shannon who will "listen" and then *proceed to write* as she has done here and instruct the rest of us in how to become connoisseurs, savants, scholars of living on this horribly polluted, plundered planet.

Shannon, in *Good Health in a Toxic World*, offers us *the* "technologic fix"—*the right use of nature*—to bring us to health. It is not a quick fix (although it *begins* at once) but it is the only one that works and that endures. This because Mother Nature will come to your rescue if you will but permit Her to do so.

—DAN ROEHM, M.D., F.A.C.P.
The Institute of Natural Medicine
Pompano Beach, Florida

INTRODUCTION

*T*hey can destroy the cell wall, destroy DNA, damage digestive enzymes, and deform brain, pancreas, and liver cells. They may contribute to heart disease, cancer, chronic fatigue syndrome, age spots, wrinkles, fatigue, and early aging. They are made as a by-product of your body's metabolism. They are usually kept in check by special enzymes and nutrients, but when there is excess chemical, radiation, or other stress, this balance is overwhelmed, and these chemical fragments take over and do their damage.

These small structures are called free radicals, and understanding their impact presents a new theory of health and disease. Although free radicals were discovered in the 1940s, and came to public attention in the late 1980s, they are still not familiar to many people. It is crucial to your health to understand free radicals and their damage potential, so you will be equipped to know how to avoid and counteract them as the newly understood way to maintain optimum health.

Free radicals are a by-product of normal metabolism—

but the *excess* free radicals, which are what concern us, are caused by toxins recently introduced to our earth, in particular man-made radiation and chemicals. So free radicals are a symptom of the greater problem, *not* the problem itself.

Compartmentalized thinking brings us to the point where we need to be reminded that our health depends upon the health of the earth, and that the health of the earth depends on *our* health. It is not just a matter of exercise, fresh vegetables, and vitamin supplements that will lead us to the health potential we yearn for. It is not just a matter of defusing stress and recycling the garbage. It is not just a matter of contacting and reassuring our inner child. Our authentic health will appear when we have assured a clean sustainable earth. Whatever our immediate daily problems, all humans need to enlarge our concerns to encompass our earth support system of air, soil, food, water, and oxygen, and to make a commitment to maintain it.

Part I of this book describes free radicals and tells about their implication in major diseases. This section is included as background to verify the facts, and you may want to flip through it and go on to the practical section, Part II, with its six chapters, each focusing on one approach to fighting free radicals: nutrition, dietary supplements, exercise, stress reduction, exposure to full-spectrum light, and avoiding pollution. Part III provides complete menus utilizing health-enhancing foods. Part IV gives you an invaluable collection of resources to find materials, books, and leads to actualize your health plans.

I present this book with wishes for your good health.

Although most trees that are harvested for paper for books are replaced, there is such a need to plant and care for trees and forests that I am donating a portion of the proceeds from the sales of this book to an organization called Global ReLeaf, which works internationally to do this.

Part I

ALL ABOUT FREE RADICALS

"It isn't that they can't see the solution, they can't see the problem."
—*G. K. Chesterton*

CHAPTER 1

What Are Free Radicals?

"When the body is overwhelmed by free radicals
disease must result." —*Stephen Levine*

*N*ew paradigms, new frameworks of thought, are emerging in many domains. These evolving perspectives allow us to understand our reality from new viewpoints. They throw light on principles that already exist but have not yet been fully understood. For example, when Louis Pasteur put forth the germ theory of disease in 1890, he revolutionized previous medical thinking. Then later in his life he understood more and came to another paradigm shift, which we are just now reaching. Before his death Pasteur said: "It is not the microbe" that causes the illness, "it is the terrain." In other words, it is the condition of the human body that determines whether the germ will have any effect on it or not.

Good Health in a Toxic World explores a new paradigm for the study of health and youth extension: the effect free radicals have on your health. This new way of understanding provides a holistic view to regaining and maintaining optimum, abundant health. Free radicals, submicroscopic chemical frag-

3

ments formed as the by-product of normal metabolism, damage the body in many ways, and sometimes the damage is severe enough to allow diseases to take hold. By learning how to counteract the influences of free radicals you can enhance your well-being and increase your longevity by fending off all of the most common illnesses, stopping the process of the symptoms of aging, and generally reinforcing overall health.

▲

"Aging at the biochemical level is based on the production of free radicals."
—BRIAN LIEBOVITZ, PH.D., "Aspects of Free Radical Reactions in Biological Systems: Aging," *Journal of Gerontology*, 1980, Vol. 35

▲

The first section of this book will explain what free radicals are, what causes them, and what damage they can do. The six chapters in Part II provide information on how to keep them in balance so they do not become overwhelming and destructive. With a section of seasonal menus to help you put healthful eating at the center of your prevention plan, and an extensive resources section, you will be equipped to benefit from this new knowledge and become the healthiest, most vigorous, and youthful self you can be.

Up until the discovery of microbes and the germ theory of Pasteur in the late nineteenth century, infectious diseases such as tuberculosis and pneumonia were responsible for most deaths. The development of antibiotics in the 1940s meant many infections could be controlled. Now degenerative diseases, heart disease, and cancer have emerged as the major causes of death, accounting for 75 percent in 1990. Compounding this shift, the ailments centering on weak immunity, including allergies, environmental illnesses, AIDS, and chronic fatigue syndrome, are now further reducing the general level of health to a point where many people complain of early aging, fatigue, memory loss, or allergies, and only a small percentage of people of any age are experiencing their full inborn vibrant health potential. *Why is this?*

▲

"Today it seems very likely that the assumption that there is a basic cause of aging is correct and that the sum of the deleterious free radical reactions going on continuously throughout the cells and tissues is the aging process or a major contributor to it."
—DENHAM HARMAN, "Free Radicals and the Origin, Evolution and Present Status of the Free Radical Theory of Aging," *Free Radicals in Molecular Biology Aging and Disease,* 1984

▲

The answer to the question *why* there is such an underpar state of health nationally—even globally—is that the production of free radicals has gotten out of control. The body produces a certain amount of free radicals as a matter of course. But in today's world, stress, pollution, and poor nutrition force overproduction of free radicals, in numbers that overwhelm the body's natural defenses against the damage they can cause. This book represents a holistic view, rather than a look at separate parts, of our current planetary and health picture.

▲

"Free radicals, highly reactive chemicals believed to have given rise to life on earth, are now increasingly regarded as primary forces of

destruction and death in nearly all living things.''
—Jane Brody, "Natural Chemicals Now Called Major Cause of Disease," *The New York Times*, April 26, 1988

▲

WHAT ARE FREE RADICALS?

The free radical is a molecule with an imbalance in electrons. All living and nonliving things are made up of units of matter called atoms. When atoms join together they are called molecules. The atom is made up of two basic parts: the nucleus and the electrons. The nucleus has a positive electric charge that balances the negative electric charge of the electrons. The electrons are arranged in pairs. There is a dynamic balance both between the pairs of electrons and between the electrons and the nucleus.

When an electron is added or removed this balance is lost, and the atom or molecule seeks to regain this balance by taking an electron from another atom.

Free Radicals Are Formed as a By-product of Metabolism
Metabolism is basically the interaction of the oxygen you breathe and the foods you eat. It is how your body generates energy and heat and disposes of carbon dioxide. Free radicals form as a natural by-product of this process. When an oxygen molecule is used to facilitate the digestion of food to produce energy, the reaction adds an electron to the molecule. This leaves an unpaired electron in the oxygen molecule and an imbalance between the nucleus and the electrons. Once this happens the oxygen becomes volatile and finds an electron to use to stabilize itself: it steals an electron from another atom

or molecule and leaves it, in turn, out of balance. This can cause a chain reaction, a self-multiplying firestorm that results in enormous cellular damage.

FOOD + OXYGEN = CARBON DIOXIDE
+
WATER
+
ENERGY
+
FREE RADICALS

▲

"The further along we get, the more we are overwhelmed by the number of disease states that involve free radicals."
—J. M. McCORD, M.D., Biochemist,
Canadian Journal of Physiological Pharmacology, 1982

▲

Aside from the destructive effects of free radicals that this book focuses on, free radicals also perform many essential functions in the body. The immune system uses them to mop up unwanted bacteria, viruses, and other potentially damaging entities such as cancer cells. Free radicals also help to generate energy the cells use, and assist in the creation of hormones and in the synthesis of proteins and nucleic acids.

While free radicals are formed in the normal metabolism process, they are also created by other influences on the body such as radiation, chemicals, cosmic rays, and ultraviolet light, which are all good at knocking electrons loose from their orbits. The most common atom that creates free radicals in humans is oxygen—and then the process is known as oxidation (the same process that causes rust, or the browning of a cut

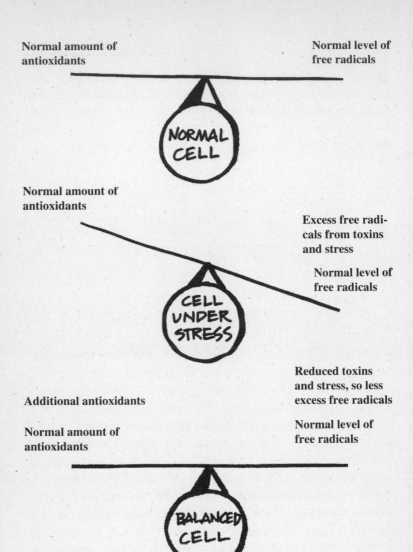

Normal amount of antioxidants

Normal level of free radicals

NORMAL CELL

Normal amount of antioxidants

Excess free radicals from toxins and stress

Normal level of free radicals

CELL UNDER STRESS

Additional antioxidants

Reduced toxins and stress, so less excess free radicals

Normal amount of antioxidants

Normal level of free radicals

BALANCED CELL

In the normal cell (top) balance is maintained. Normal levels of free radicals are neutralized by antioxidant enzymes and antioxidants. In the cell under stress (center) the excess free radicals create imbalance and disease. In the balanced cell (bottom) the environmental toxins are reduced, and the addition of antioxidants and antioxidant enzymes restores balance.

apple). In normal circumstances, the body neutralizes free radicals with antioxidants—the most familiar ones are vitamins C, E, and A. It is only when too many stress factors cause *excess* free radicals, and antioxidants become overwhelmed, that free radicals start to wreak havoc on your health.

▲

"Everything is the way it is because we are
the way we are."
—CHRISTOPHER HILLS, *Rise of the Phoenix*,
1979.

▲

OXYGEN AND ANTIOXIDANTS

Three to four billion years ago the earth's atmosphere had no oxygen. When an early life form, algae, developed, it lived on sunlight and water and released oxygen. The oxygen formed supported the development of life as we now know it. It also made the protective ozone layer surrounding the earth, which allowed a variety of life-forms to develop. These early life-forms had to contend with free radicals as a by-product of oxygen metabolism, and needed to counteract their damage in order to survive. A mechanism to do this evolved through the development of enzymes created in the body specifically for this purpose, and through the use of antioxidant nutrients. A balance thus emerged between the destructive aspect of oxygen-based metabolism and the antioxidant enzymes and nutrients used to neutralize its damage.

Your body is about 75 percent water. Water is approximately eight ninths oxygen. So overall your body is approximately two thirds oxygen. Oxygen is essential: without it body cells would die in a few minutes. The word "antioxidant" could give the impression that oxygen is the problem, but don't let that fool you. The excess production of free radicals is the problem.

Currently, our oxygen resources are low on earth. The percentage of oxygen in the air is down to about 19 percent. Some experts say that we may have originally evolved in an atmosphere of 38 percent oxygen. But now, due to the loss of forests and ocean plankton, our two major sources of oxygen production, measurements of oxygen as low as 12 percent and 15 percent have been made in heavily industrialized areas. This oxygen-depleted condition is a contributing cause of the generalized lack of well-being that many are experiencing.

▲

"Even when the evidence suggests that free radicals are not totally responsible for a particular disease entity, their involvement often seems to play a part in the disease process."
—PETER SOUTHERN, "Free Radicals in Medicine," *Mayo Clinic Proceedings* 63, 1988

▲

WHAT CAUSES FREE RADICALS?

The excess production of free radicals occurs when the body is subjected to chemicals, radiation, and psychological stress. The following pages provide a summary of some of the extraordinary free-radical-causing stresses of modern life, and at the end of the chapter you will find documenting references. This is just a brief outline. Part II discusses in depth how these stresses cause the creation of excess free radicals, how those free radicals cause health problems, and how to protect yourself from these various influences.

Air Quality

Ultraviolet Rays

Family

Emotion

Work

Stress

Mental Attitude

Light

Noise

Chemicals

Radiation

Water Quality

Food Quality

▲

"In 1990 we have 100,000 percent more chemicals on our farm products than we did in 1945."
—JOHN ROBBINS, *Our Food, Our World*, 1992

▲

Pollutants

The last fifty or so years have been characterized by the release of tens of thousands of man-made chemicals into our environment. Between the years 1965 and 1978, over 4 million new chemical compounds were reported. About 60,000 chemicals are in common use today, many of whose toxicity is not known.

▲

"High Levels of Lead Found in Water Serving 30 Million"
—*The New York Times*, May 12, 1992

▲

Drinking water can hardly retain that adjective, unless you want to add to your toxic load. Water is one of the major ways our bodies are exposed to toxins. Twenty-some chemicals are intentionally added to water allegedly to make it drinkable—including fluoride, which is in 60 percent of U.S. water, chlorine, which is in all water, and aluminum, which is in most water. Aside from these known toxins, runoff from chemicals put on crops, and radioactive fallout from the nuclear industry go into groundwater and reservoirs. These are serious reasons for you to take steps to assure a clean water supply for you and your family.

Air Pollution

Air pollution is another main source of exposure to toxins. Millions of tons of toxic pollutants are released into the atmosphere each year in the United States. Especially when concentrated in urban areas, these toxins react with oxygen in the presence of sunlight to form photochemical smog, which when inhaled causes free radicals and immune system suppression. (See Chapter 8 for more details.)

Cigarette Smoke

We well know about the hazards of tar and nicotine from smoking cigarettes. What is rarely mentioned is the fact that cigarette smoke reacts in the body to create free radicals, which is what can lead to lung fibrosis, emphysema, and cancer. In addition, the Surgeon General's 1979 *Report on Smoking and Health* reports that cigarettes contain radioactive polonium, and this toxin is a prime element in causing tobacco's damage.

Stress

Stress generates high levels of adrenaline and other body chemicals, which result in an increased production of free radicals. Modern life presents many occasions for stress, so there may be almost constant production of stress-related free radicals.

Excess Exercise

Exercise in itself is a cause of free radicals but your body can normally handle these. *Excess* exercise, which is a lot more than your daily visit to the gym or an afternoon hike, is known to cause excess free radicals. Here it is a matter of balance. Exercise is necessary and health-building; too much weakens the body through the formation of excess free radicals. Athletes in training often counteract this with extra free radical fighters.

▲

"Splitting the atom; uncontrollable emission of radioactive toxins; the insanity of the nuclear, bacteriological and chemical weapons build-up;

unrestrained economic growth spreading
commercialization to every aspect of our lives;
overconsumption of goods and raw materials;
anti-human architecture, transport, technology
and food production—these are the conditions
of modern industrial society, and these are the
factors responsible for disease.''
—PETRA KELLY, *Fighting for Hope*, 1984

▲

Radiation

Denham Harman did his research on free radical formation in the 1950s using radiation as the cause of the free radicals. Since the work of Abram Petkau in 1972, it is known
that low doses of radiation cause physiological damage through
the formation of free radicals. Radiation sickness is a disease
caused by the unleashing of excess free radicals in the body.
In high doses, like the Hiroshima bomb blast, radiation causes
damage to the nucleus of the atom, bypassing the electrons. In
contrast, low doses knock the electrons out of the atom, causing the generation of free radicals. So the everyday amount of
radiation that is released as part of the normal operation of the
world's 400 nuclear power plants (about 110 in the United
States) is of grave concern. Nuclear power plants must have
releases in order to function, and these releases, even though
they may be partially filtered, allow radiation to go into your
air and water, and onto farmland and into your food. (See
Chapter 8 for more on this, and the references for reading on
this critical subject in Part IV.)

With high-altitude jet travel, which is usually about
30,000 feet or six miles, you are exposed to cosmic rays that
cause free radicals. It is thought by some that jet lag may be

mostly a fatigue brought about by this exposure to excess free radicals and not so much the result of "meridian hopping."

▲

"The induction of immuno suppression by UV-B has now been demonstrated in humans."
—*Environmental Effects of Ozone Depletion*, Executive Summary by the United Nations Environment Program, November 1991

▲

Ultraviolet Rays

Until recently ozone in the stratosphere acted as a filter for damaging ultraviolet rays. Now with the combination of chemicals and radioactive releases the ozone loss over the United States is proceeding twice as fast as predicted when awareness of this problem first emerged in the late 1980s. The National Aeronautics and Space Administration (NASA) and the National Oceanic and Atmospheric Administration recorded the most dangerously depleted levels of ozone in history over the United States in the spring of 1993. The ultraviolet rays, especially ones such as UV-B that were previously kept by the ozone layer from reaching earth, are known to be free radical generators. (There is a discussion of this in Chapter 7.)

▲

"By deliberately changing their image of reality people are changing the world."
—WILLIS HARMAN, *Global Mind Change*, 1990

▲

HOW EXCESS FREE RADICALS DAMAGE HEALTH

Uncontrolled free radicals damage body cells either by breaking down the cell membrane, by attacking the internal working of the cell, or by going right to the nucleus to attack the genetic material. A fundamental way that free radicals cause their damage is by breaking down natural body fats. Since the cell membrane is composed of fatty tissue (called lipids), it is a target for free radical attack. They may destroy the cell membrane, so that it cannot take in nutrients or release wastes. This leads eventually to the collapse and death of the cell.

Free radicals can damage white blood cells and particularly the defender T cells, both of which are key to a strong immune system—and enable you to ward off bacteria and viruses. Free radicals may also weaken essential antibodies that are produced by the immune system to protect from disease, resulting in susceptibility to communicable diseases. Uncontrolled free radicals may disturb nerve chemicals, which can affect the brain and nervous system. They may slow or distort the transmission of messages by damaging neurotransmitters, resulting in memory loss and mental problems including senile dementia. Free radicals may also eat away at the protective myelin sheath around the nerves, limiting reflexes or causing multiple sclerosis.

Digestive enzymes are also vulnerable to free radical assault, reducing their ability to digest and utilize food and thus limiting the absorption of nutrients.

Free radicals may injure the lubricating synovial fluid around the joints, causing inflammation and pain and resulting in arthritis, bursitis, or gout.

▲

"The antioxidant defense system is, of course,
finite in its capacity to resist oxidative stress—
when the body is overwhelmed by excess
oxidative stress disease must result."
—STEPHEN LEVINE, *Oxidative Adaptation*,
1986

▲

Free radicals cause what science calls "cross-linking," a
hooking together of cell structures that may be partly responsible for hardening of the arteries, stiffness of joints, and wrinkling of skin—many of the manifestations of what is referred
to as aging. Cross-linking in the lungs causes emphysema.

Free radicals may damage genes, the DNA and RNA in
the cell nucleus that mastermind the creation of new cells.
When a cell with a damaged gene divides to make two cells,
the new cell may be abnormal. When the DNA is damaged it
tends to reproduce new cells very rapidly—the hallmark of
what we call cancer. Damaged DNA may produce cells that
are not able to function as they were meant to, resulting in,
for example, deterioration of tissue and organs and messenger
hormones, among many other things.

Free radicals account for nearly all of the signs and symptoms we think of as normal (and inevitable) in aging. An article
in the August 1992 issue of the journal *Science* centers on "the
importance of free radical damage to nucleic acids and lipids
in age-related disease processes." It explains what a difficult
task the human body faces in counteracting free radicals, which
some researchers believe are responsible for 10,000 or so alterations to the DNA *per cell per day*. The article concludes, a
"fraction of such a massive amount of damage would escape
repairs by even the most sophisticated mechanisms and the

accumulation of unrepaired damage could account for the age-related loss of physiological function.''

In an overall sense, free radicals can also cause malformed molecules—which the immune system sees as foreign invaders. The immune system reacts to clear them out, eventually becoming worn down and exhausted in the process—and unable to fully combat the real enemies it faces. This then allows disease to take hold where it could not have been able to if the immune system were not overburdened. The weakest points start to go first. In one person it may be arthritis, in another it may be extreme fatigue, in another allergies, and so on.

▲

''Under pathological conditions much larger amounts of free radicals are formed than normal and these can overwhelm the defenses of the cell and lead to damage and even death of the cell.''
—PETER SOUTHERN and GARTH POWIS, *Free Radicals in Medicine*, 1988

▲

Free radical damage to cells progresses to tissues and organs and results principally in heart disease, cancer, diabetes, arthritis, and diseases of immune suppression.

In brief, free radicals can damage any organ system of the body. When we see these effects as laymen, we pass them off as ''aging''; medical scientists now term these phenomena as ''degenerative diseases.''

TOXIN > FREE RADICAL > CELL DAMAGE > TISSUE DAMAGE >
DISEASE

THE IMMUNE SYSTEM AND AUTOIMMUNE DISEASES

The immune system is the body's protective system, which has the purpose of ensuring survival of the individual. It does this by looking out for any alien structures, and when it sees them, it engulfs and removes them. It is composed of a network or organs, hormones, and special cells that defend the body from bacteria, virus, and cancer cells by neutralizing them.

There are about a trillion lymphocytes, white blood cells, which become differentiated by the immune system to do different jobs. The thymus gland is where white blood cells are turned into T cells. The thymus is vulnerable to free radical damage, thus affecting its function of creating T cells from white blood cells.

EXCESS FREE RADICALS EXHAUST THE IMMUNE SYSTEM

The function of the immune system is to distinguish what should be there from what should not be there. It has the brilliant ability to differentiate between what is a part of the body and what is an alien invader. This alien might be a germ from outside, or one of your own cells turned malignant. Or it could be a malformed structure caused by a free radical reaction. Mopping up too many of these odd structures will weaken the immune system.

The Parts of the Immune System

The immune system has three functions:

1. It concentrates the antigens (bacteria, etc. that are alien to the body) into a few places—spleen and lymph nodes.
2. It circulates white blood cells and T cells through these places.
3. It produces cells specifically made to get rid of these antigens.

The Immune System Declines By:

1. Passive wearing out when it is overloaded with excess free radicals.
2. Active self-destruction when it attacks itself.

When immune cells such as lymphocytes or T cells are weakened by free radicals they may fail to distinguish friend or foe. So they may attack cells that they mistake as foreign, while, in fact, damaging the body's own cells; this behavior results in what is called an autoimmune disease.

SOME AUTOIMMUNE DISEASES	TARGET
Addison's disease	Adrenal gland
Autoimmune hemolytic anemia	Red blood cell membrane proteins
Crohn's disease	Gut
Graves' disease	Thyroid
Hashimoto's thyroiditis	Thyroid
Idiopathic thrombocytopenic purpura	Platelets
Insulin-dependent diabetes	Pancreatic cells

Some Autoimmune Diseases	Target
Pernicious anemia	Gastric parietal cells
Psoriasis	Skin
Systemic lupus erythematosus	DNA, blood cells, other tissues

The upsetting of nature's balancing ways through pollution contributes to the production of *excess* free radicals. Free radicals are a major cause of human health problems and they, in turn, are a result of the overall health problem of the toxic earth. The earth is our life-support system, offering air and water and food to sustain us. As this ecosystem deteriorates the amount of free radicals generated increases. Because so many ecological and medical issues have been viewed in a fragmented and compartmentalized way, the relationship between our planet and our health has not been clearly presented. It is only when too many stress factors cause *excess* free radicals and the antioxidant defenses become overwhelmed that we find an increased incidence of early aging and disease. The following chapter discusses free-radical-related health problems with documentation from medical literature. Part II then goes into practical pointers as to what we can do to safeguard our own health and the health of our habitat, the earth.

RESOURCES: FREE RADICALS

Aging

"The Free Radical Theory of Aging: Advances in Free Radical Biology and Medicine"
R.J. Melhorn and G. Cole
Advances in Free Radical Biology and Medicine, 1:165–223, 1985

"Protein Oxidation and Aging"
R.R. Stadtman
Science, August 28, 1992

Free Radical Theory of Aging: A Theory Based on Free Radical and Radiation Chemistry
Denham Harman, M.D.
University of California Radiation Lab Report, No. 378, July 14, 1955

"Role of Free Radicals: Aging and Disease"
Denham Harman, M.D.
In *Relations Between Normal Aging and Disease*,
ed. H.A. Johnson, Raven Press, NY, 1984, pp. 78–82

"The Role of Oxygen Free Radicals in Human Disease
Processes"
G.B. Bulkley
Surgery 94:407–11, 1983

"DNA Damage and Free Radicals"
O.I. Aruoma and B. Halliwell
Chem. BR 149–51, 1991

"Oxygen Free Radicals Linked to Many Diseases"
Jean Marx
Science 235:528–31, Jan. 30, 1987

Oxygen

"Beyond Antioxidant Adaptation: A Free Radical Hypoxia-
Clonal Thesis of Cancer Causation"
Levine and Kidd
Journal of Orthomolecular Medicine 14(3):189–213,
1985

The Prime Cause of Cancer, 1969.
O. Warburg
1966 Lindau Lecture, English edition by D. Burk,
Wurzburg, Germany, K. Triltsch

"Metabolic Abnormalities in Patients with Chronic
Candidiasis: The Acetyldehyde Hypothesis"
O.C. Truss
Journal of Orthomolecular Medicine 13(2), 1984

Oxygen Therapies: A New Way of Looking at Disease
E. McCabe
Available from Energy Publications, 4-RD1, Morrisville, NJ 13408

Sauerstoffkrise (Oxygen Crisis)
Hans Bassfeld
This book (in German only) documenting the oxygen drop over Europe is available from Ingenieurburo fur Umweltfragen, Gleiwitzer Strasse 4, 4220 Dinslaken, Germany; tel: (01234) 55488

Pollutants

"Free Radical Intermediates in the Metabolism of Toxic Chemicals"
R.P. Mason
In *Free Radicals in Biology*, ed., W.A. Pryor
Vol. 5, New York Academic Press, 1983, pp. 163–221

"Free Radical Biology: Xenobiotics, Cancer and Aging"
W.A. Pryor
New York Academy of Science Annals, Vol. 393, 1982

"Mechanisms of Chemical Toxicity—A Unifying Hypothesis"
D.V. Parke
Regul Pharmacol Toxicol 2:267–86, 1982

"Toxicant-Disease-Environment Interactions Associated with Suppression of the Immune System, Growth and Reproduction"
W.P. Porter
Science 224:1014–17, June 1, 1984

"Chemical Sensitivity: Breaking the Paralyzing Paradigm"
  Sherry Rogers
  Internal Medicine Report, pp. 8–31, March 15, 1992
  This article explains how chemically triggered free
  radicals cause tissue damage. There are 102 references
  Available from Dr. Sherry Rogers, P.O. Box 3161,
  Syracuse, NY 13220

"Carcinogenesis, Vascular Disease, and the Free Radical
  Reaction"
  F.C. Johnson
  Nutrition and Cancer 3:117–21, 1982

"Ground Water Contamination in the United States"
  V. Pye
  Science 221:713–18, 1983

Fluoride: The Aging Factor
  John Yiamouyannis
  Health Action Press, Delaware, OH, 1983

Fluoridation: The Great Dilemma
  George Waldbott
  Coronado Press, Lawrence, KS, 1978

Cigarette Smoke

"Oxygen Radicals and Air Pollution. Oxidative Stress:
  Oxidants and Anti-Oxidants"
  S. Hippeli
  Inst Fur Botanik U Microbiologie, Munich, Germany,
  Chapters 3–55, 1991

"On Anti-Oxidant Nutrients: How They Protect You from
  Smog and Other Environmental Pollutants and Some
  Aging Reactions"
  A.L. Tappel
  Executive Health Magazine, 1980

"Singlet Oxygen Production from the Reaction of Ozone with Biological Molecules"
J.R. Kanofsky et al.
Journal of Biological Chemistry, 266:9039–42, 1991

The Free Radical Chemistry of Cigarette Smoke and Its Toxicological Implications
D.F. Church and W.A. Pryor
Environmental Health Perspectives, 1984

The Health Consequences of Smoking: A Report of the Surgeon General
United States Office on Smoking and Health
U.S. Government Printing Office, Washington, DC 20402, 1983

"Ionizing Radiation from Tobacco"
J.B. Westin
Journal of the American Medical Association, pp. 257–2169, 1987

"The Role of Free Radicals in Human Disease"
G.B. Bulkley
Surgery, Sept. 1983

Stress

Understanding Allergy, Sensitivity and Immunity
J.V. Ionega
Rutgers University Press, 1990, pp. 266–70

"Stress-Mechanisms of Immunosuppression"
J.E. Dohms
Veterinary Immunology and Immunopathology
30:89–109, 1991

"Interactions Between the Immune System and the Nervous System"
R.E. Faith et al.
In *Stress and Immunity*, N. Plotnikoff et al., eds.
CRC Press, Boca Raton, 1991, pp. 287–304

Antioxidant Adaptation: Its Role in Free Radical Pathology
S. Levine and P. Kidd
Allergy Research Group, San Leandro, CA, 1986

Radiation

Diet for the Atomic Age
Sara Shannon
Avery Publishing Group, 1987
See pp. 6–10 concerning cosmic rays

"Free Radicals, Antioxidants and Human Disease"
Barry Halliwell et al.
Journal of Laboratory and Clinical Medicine, June 1992, pp. 598–620
See p. 602 concerning free radicals and exercise

The Chemical Basis of Radiation Biology
C. Von Sonntag
Taylor and Francis, London, 1987

"Effects of 22Na+ on a Phospholipid Membrane"
Abram Petkau
Health Physics 22:239–44, 1972

Radiation Induced Cancer from Low Dose Exposure
John Gofman, M.D., Ph.D.
Committee for Nuclear Responsibility, San Francisco, 1991

Jet Travel

Radiation Exposure of Air Carrier Crewmembers
FAA, U.S. Department of Transportation, AAM-6624,
March 5, 1990

Understanding In-Flight Radiation
R.J. Barish, Ph.D.
In-Flight Radiation Protection Services, New York, NY
10021
April 1989, p. 55

Jet Smart
Diana Fairchild
Flyana Rhyme Inc., Maui, HI, 1992

Ultraviolet Rays

"Protection Against Ultraviolet Radiation"
Abram Hoffer
Canadian Medical Association Journal 147:839–40, Sept.
15, 1992

"Skin Cancer Rate in Battered Kauai on the Rise"
John Dinolfo
Medical Tribune, October 8, 1992, p. 32

Bob Worrest, Ph.D.
Address at the International Conference on Ozone
Depletion and Ultraviolet Impacts, Whistler, B.C.
Canada, September 22–24, 1993
Proceedings of this conference available from Air Waste
Management Association (412) 232-3444

Disease and Aging

"Free Radicals, Anti-Oxidants and Human Disease"
Barry Halliwell et al.
Journal of Laboratory and Clinical Medicine,
119:598–620, June 1992

Article is available from Dr. B. Halliwell, Pulmonary-Critical Care Medicine, UC Davis Professional Building, 4301 X Street, Room 2120, Sacramento, CA 958217

"Oxygen Free Radicals Linked to Many Diseases"
Jean Marx
Science 235:529, January 30, 1987

"Free Radicals in Medicine: Involvement in Human Disease"
Peter Southern
Mayo Clinic Proceedings 63:390–408, 1988

Free Radicals in Biology and Medicine
Barry Halliwell and John Gotteridge
Clarendon Press, Oxford, 1989

"The Role of Oxygen Free Radicals in Human Disease Processes"
G.B. Bulkely
Surgery 94:407–11, 1983

"Dietary Carcinogens and Anticarcinogens: Oxygen Radicals and Degenerative Diseases"
Bruce Ames
Science 23:1256–63, 1983

"DNA Damage and Free Radicals"
O.I. Arouma and B. Halliwell
Chem BR, 1991, pp. 149–51

"Protein Oxidation and Aging"
E.R. Stadtman
Science, Aug. 28, 1992

Journal of the American Medical Association, Vol. 268, Nov. 25, 1992
This entire issue is on the immune link to disease

"The Free Radical Theory of Aging"
R.J. Melhorn and G. Cole
Advances in Free Radical Biology and Medicine
I:165–223, 1985

"Age Related Change in Thymus"
K. Hirokawa
Acta Pathologica, Japan 28:843–57, 1978

CHAPTER 2
Major Diseases Connected to Free Radical Damage

"In the face of sustained oxidative stress, the organism's antioxidant defenses may be taxed beyond their capabilities; the likely consequences are chronic degenerative changes."
—*Stephen Levine*

*M*ore than 6,000 scientific articles on free radicals testify to the fact that free radicals contribute to many major diseases. One of these, "Oxygen Free Radicals Linked to Many Diseases" (Marx 1987), declares: "Oxygen free radicals may contribute to the development or exacerbation of many of mankind's most common ills including cancer, heart attacks, stroke, emphysema." Researcher G.B. Bulkley points out in "The Role of Oxygen Free Radicals in Human Disease Processes" (*Surgery*, September 1983): "Free radical injury may play a role in a wide range of disease processes. They are the primary means by which radiation injures tissue, and by which many drugs, carcinogens and other toxic agents exert their effects."

Scientists and researchers around the world agree that free-radical-generated loss of cell membrane integrity compromises cellular function, damages enzymes, and that the constant aggravation to the immune system from free radical assaults causes it to deteriorate, resulting in the loss of youth-fulness and the possibility of disease.

What follows is a discussion of the major degenerative diseases, the number of people who suffer from them in the United States, and how they correlate with excess free radical production. Articles from medical journals supporting the free radical implication in disease states are at the end of this section.

▲

"Of course our failures are a consequence of many factors, but possibly one of the most important is the fact that society operates on the theory that specialisation is the key to success, not realising that specialisation precludes comprehensive thinking."
—R. BUCKMINSTER FULLER, *Operating Manual for Spaceship Earth*, 1969

▲

CANCER

Estimated number of new cancer cases in 1993 totaled 1,170,000.
—American Cancer Society

497,000 Americans died of cancer in 1989, the most recent year for statistics.
—1993 *Information Please Almanac*

In 1900 cancer accounted for 4 percent of deaths in the United States. It is now the second leading cause of death.
> —Judith Brady, 1993
> *One in Three Women with Cancer*, Cleis Press

In 1980 a woman's risk of breast cancer was 1 in 11; in 1991, 1 in 9; in June 1993, the risk is 1 in 8.
> —American Cancer Society

In 1990, 1 in 3 Americans will develop cancer and the number will double in the 1990s.
> —*Meditrends 1991–1992.*
> A report from the American Hospital Association

▲

"We have come to view cancer susceptibility as a direct consequence of exhaustion of the antioxidant defense system. In this context, exposure to antioxidant chemicals; irradiation damage; emotional stress, all are potentially oncogenic [cancer-forming]."
> —STEPHEN LEVINE, *Antioxidant Adaptation*, 1986

▲

In the initial stage of cancer, a physical, chemical, or biological agent (including free radicals) causes an alteration in the structure of the DNA, the chromosomes that carry the genetic blueprint, resulting in incorrect structure of new cells. When the DNA is damaged it tends to reproduce new cells incorrectly and very rapidly—becoming what we call cancer. Depending on where it is located, it may be called liver cancer, bone cancer, or breast cancer, or one of many others.

The immune system is ever alert to catch this syndrome,

but when it has already been weakened by overwork in reacting to free-radical-generated malformed cells, it cannot function up to its potential, and the result is cancer. Presumably, up to some point in this process, it could be interrupted or corrected by the reduction of exposure to carcinogens and/or an increase in free radical fighters.

▲

"It is only by repairing the damage we have done to the natural world that we can recreate conditions in which the incidence of these diseases can be reduced to a minimum."
—Edward Goldsmith, *The Way: An Ecological World View*, 1993

▲

One of the many research papers connecting free radical damage and cancer appeared in the journal *Cancer Research* in 1991. The authors, Donald Malins and Russom Haimanot, report that in breast cancer, the hydroxyl radical (a type of free radical) "produces alterations in the structural integrity of DNA bases. Unless the modified DNA is promptly repaired, miscoding may occur in replication which may result in the formation of" cancerous cells.

According to a 1990 General Accounting Office report (GAO-T-PEMD) titled *Radiation Induced Cancers*, the likelihood is increasing that a woman will be diagnosed with breast cancer at some point in her lifetime, and concludes that there has been no progress in preventing the disease. It is apparent that traditional approaches aren't working, but an understanding of free radical damage suggests a new path. Because cancer-producing agents exert their effect via free radical formation, searching out the sources of free radicals in women's environment could be fruitful in finding a cause of this increase in breast cancer.

▲

"During the past two decades an ever-increasing body of knowledge has implicated free radical mediated processes in a wide spectrum of different types of human disease."
—PETER SOUTHERN AND GARTH POWIS,
"Free Radicals in Medicine," *Mayo Clinic Proceedings* 63, 1988

▲

HEART DISEASE

Nearly 69 million people, more than 1 in 4, suffer from some form of cardiovascular disease.
—1993 *Information Please Almanac*

50 million have hypertension.
—National Heart, Lung and Blood Institute, 1992

6 million have chronic heart disease.
—National Heart, Lung and Blood Institute, 1985

7 million have coronary heart disease.
—National Heart, Lung and Blood Institute, 1992

2.5 million have cerebrovascular disease.
—National Heart, Lung and Blood Institute, 1985

2.5 million have hardening of the arteries.
—National Heart, Lung and Blood Institute, 1985

Approximately 700,000 heart attack victims are admitted to hospitals every year.
—*Science*, January 30, 1987

▲

"Emancipate yourself from mental slavery."
—BOB MARLEY, Musician

▲

For all the talk about cholesterol as the cause of heart disease, many recent studies point to excess free radicals as the real cause. Free radicals cause damage to the walls of arteries, resulting in plaques, and they also change cholesterol chemistry. The combination of the two results in atherosclerosis, which in turn can cause heart attack (or a stroke). Plaque formation in arteries is not caused by high levels of cholesterol alone. The type of cholesterol known as the HDL form, or the "good" cholesterol, has the ability to quench free radicals. In this process, the good form of HDL cholesterol turns into the "bad" form of cholesterol—LDL. In response, the immune system engages scavenger cells to remove the LDL cholesterol and in so doing they both may get stuck on the walls of the artery, where they snag other sticky platelets in the blood. All this results in the plaques, which inhibit blood transport.

Thus a high level of "bad" cholesterol molecules is an index of how many free radicals you have had to neutralize with your good HDL cholesterol. Although LDL cholesterol is viewed as "bad," it is really the result of the protective action of HDL cholesterol. So, in fact, cholesterol is a great free radical scavenger, contrary to all the negative news we've heard about it over the last few years. The focus should shift from the cholesterol itself to the excess free radicals that it mops up, thus creating the "bad" form, which in turn creates plaques in the arteries.

▲

"In our every deliberation, we must consider the impact of our decisions on the next seven generations."
—The Great Law of the Iroquois Confederacy

▲

ARTHRITIS

37 million people have arthritis.
—National Center for Health Statistics, 1992

Arthritis is characterized by swelling of joints, especially knees, fingers, and elbows. Synovial fluid, which surrounds the joints, becomes inflamed, creating a cascade of free radicals, which in turn damage the joints, breaking down collagen and connective tissue.

DIABETES

Over 14 million people have diabetes, the fourth leading cause of death.
—American Diabetes Association, 1993

Many researchers now agree than the cells in the pancreas that are responsible for making insulin can be damaged by free radicals—the end result being diabetes. A high-sugar, low-fiber diet and inadequate minerals are the other major contributing causes of diabetes. A low-sugar, high-fiber diet and adequate minerals are effective in controlling the disease because it gives forth fewer free radicals to contend with. This explains why there are no particular anti-cancer, anti-heart disease, anti-arthritis diets anymore—they are all the same. All are anti–free radical diets.

MENTAL DISORDERS

There are approximately 4 million cases of Alzheimer's disease.
—Alzheimer's Association, 1993

Over 10 million Americans may suffer from depression.
—Pfizer U.S. Pharmaceuticals Company, 1993

38 million Americans suffer from some sort of mental illness.
—Mental Illness Foundation, 1993

4 million people, between 15 and 30 years of age, experience schizophrenia.
—Mental Illness Foundation, 1993

New research indicates that free radicals can damage brain cells and neurotransmitters, and they are implicated in schizophrenia, autism, Alzheimer's disease, and Down's syndrome. Free radicals caused by exposure to radiation are implicated in lowered intelligence. Research by Dr. Ernest Sternglass revealed lower SAT college test scores among students born at the time of atmospheric bomb testing with its widespread radioactive fallout, 1955 to 1963. Test scores of those born before 1955 and after 1963 were higher, showing that the drop was not due to television or frozen food. Dr. Harmon, the father of the free radical theory of aging, proposes that Alzheimer's disease is explained in part by free radical damage.

▲

"If a man walks in the woods for love of them
half each day, he is in danger of being
regarded as a loafer; but if he spends his whole
day as a speculator, shearing off those woods
and making earth bald before him, he is
esteemed an industrious and enterprising
citizen."
—HENRY DAVID THOREAU, "Life Without
Principle," *Atlantic Monthly*, 1863

▲

CATARACTS

Over 400,000 people a year develop cataracts.
  —Paul Jacques, *Micronutrients in Health and Disease
  on Prevention*, 1992

Cataracts, the number one cause of blindness, are caused
by free radical attack on cell membranes of the eye. Primarily
those over sixty-five usually are affected due to accumulated
free radical damage, but cataracts increasingly affect those
much younger.

ALLERGIES

Approximately 60 million Americans have allergies.
  —U.S. Department of Health and Human Services, 1992

An allergy is a response by the immune system to a
substance that is not normally harmful to it. The cells of the

immune system that identify invaders overreact to an innocuous substance, causing the allergic symptoms of stuffy nose, asthma, skin problems, or other reactions. This occurs more easily when the immune system has been compromised, as will happen as a result of an excess of free radicals.

▲

"The Time is ripe for a radical turn of events."
—JOSÉ ARGUILLES, *The Transformative Vision*, 1992

▲

ASTHMA

Over 12 million Americans suffer from asthma.
    —Centers for Disease Control, Atlanta, 1991

From 1980 to 1990 the number of reported asthma cases increased 38 percent from 6.8 million to 10.3 million. From 1980 to 1989 the death rate from asthma increased 46 percent.
    —Chronic Disease Surveillance Bureau,
        National Center for Chronic Disease Prevention
        and Health Promotion, 1991

Asthma, which involves spasm in the airways in the lungs, is usually brought on by an allergic reaction. The health of the immune system and the level of toxins that are involved determine whether or not exposure to an allergen brings on an asthma attack.

▲

"No creature, not even swine, befouls its nest
with such abandon as does homosapiens,
poisoning its habitat with fiendishly concocted
chemicals and their deadly toxic waste. A
morass of rotting human flesh awaits us all
unless the antidotes are rapidly applied."
—CHRISTOPHER BIRD, *Secrets of the Soil*,
1989

▲

MULTIPLE SCLEROSIS

There have been 150,000 to 500,000 reported cases of
multiple sclerosis since 1970. The numbers could be
much higher because multiple sclerosis is difficult to
diagnose.
—Multiple Sclerosis Association of America, 1993

Multiple sclerosis is a degenerative condition of the central nervous system. Because the myelin sheath around the
nerves deteriorates there is a progressive loss of body functions. M.S. is usually thought to be of unknown origin, although it does correlate with a weak immune system, which
mistakenly attacks this protective myelin sheath. Some researchers have found that the nerve covering is damaged by
free radicals, which in turn affects nerve conduction.

TUBERCULOSIS

27,000 cases of TB were reported in the United States in
1992. Nationally, over the past 7 years about 52,000

cases of TB have occurred above what the trend would
have predicted up to 1985.
—*The Continuing Challenge of Tuberculosis*, October 1993
    A report by the Office of Technology Assessment, Govern-
    ment Printing Office

The number of cases of TB that are resistant to antibiotics
has risen to between one quarter and one third of all
cases in New York State.
—New York State Department of Health, October 1993

One third of the world's population, 1.7 billion people,
carry the TB bacterium. It lies dormant while the
person's immune system is strong.
—*AIDS in the World: A Global Report*, 1992

Tuberculosis is a contagious disease caused by the bacteria *Mycobacterium tuberculosis*. It affects the lungs and can
be debilitating. It is known to be found among people with a
weakened immune system. An excess of free radicals may
have contributed to this reduced immunity.

An antibiotic-resistant strain of TB appeared in 1992. This
mutated bacterium was predicted in the 1950s by the Russian
physicist Andrei Sakharov, who said there would be a combination of weakened immune systems worldwide and "a global
increase in mutations of bacteria and viruses."

▲

"The earth does not belong to humans.
Humans belong to the earth. Humans do not
weave the web of life; they are merely a strand
in it. Whatever they do to the web they do to
themselves. When the thicket and the eagle
and the swift pony are gone from the land it

will mark the end of living and the beginning
of survival.''
—CHIEF SEATTLE

▲

CHRONIC FATIGUE IMMUNE DYSFUNCTION SYNDROME (CFIDS)

Also known as chronic fatigue syndrome or chronic Epstein Barr syndrome.

There are at least 1 million Americans currently carrying
a diagnosis of CFIDS and possibly another 5 million who
are ill and yet to be diagnosed.
—Dr. Hugh Fudenburg, Immunologist
February 6, 1990

''21 percent of the general population displays symptoms
of CFIDS.''
—Frequency of Chronic Active Epstein Barr Virus
Infection in a General Medical Practice''
Journal of American Medical Association, 1987

''Many people throughout the world, perhaps indeed 1
percent to 1.5 percent of all people, suffer from a
syndrome the constant feature of which is extraordinary,
almost indescribable muscle fatigue that makes even the
most minimum exercise difficult.''
—John Dwyer, M.D., Ph.D.
The Body at War, NAL Books, 1988

At least 3.5 per 100,000 people have CFIDS.
—Centers for Disease Control, Atlanta, 1992

Chronic fatigue immune dysfunction syndrome refers to a persistent and debilitating fatigue that does not resolve with bedrest and that reduces daily activity by 50 percent for at least six months. Symptoms may include fever, painful lymph nodes, muscle pain, sore throat, generalized headaches, prolonged fatigue after exercise, memory loss, and foggy mental state. CFIDS differs from environmental illness (see next section) in that the fatigue is consistent and not directly related to an immediate exposure to a chemical or other toxin. This does not mean CFIDS is not related to the overall exposure to toxins that we all experience today.

▲

"The free radical pathology which underlies
ecological illness is likely to play a primary
role in the development and metastatic spread
of many cancers, as well as in the
cardiovascular diseases, emphysema, arthritis,
cataracts and diabetes."
—STEPHEN A. LEVINE, *Antioxidant
Adaptation*, 1986

▲

ENVIRONMENTAL ILLNESS

Approximately 37 million Americans suffer from
environmental illness.
                    —National Academy of Sciences, 1987

Environmental illness occurs when the immune system is worn down by unprecedented exposure to chemicals and can no longer fulfill its function of helping the body to adapt to toxins. The result is extreme fatigue and allergic reactions.

Symptoms may include asthma, bronchitis, arthritis, fatigue, and depression.

▲

"Recent studies have suggested that free radicals can stimulate the activation (and proliferation) of HIV."
—C. SAPPEY, Grepo Laboratoire, Grenoble, France, 1993

▲

CANDIDIASIS

Approximately 60 to 70 million Americans suffer from this yeast-related condition.
—Sol Silverman, M.D., University of California, 1992

Candida albicans is a yeast normally found in the body that does not cause trouble until it overgrows. Abnormal growth is usually due to a weakened immune system, use of antibiotics, or other health-depleting situations. Candida releases toxins that further weaken immunity and result in the ailment referred to as candidiasis, or candida. The candida fungus may travel through the bloodstream to various parts of the body and result in a variety of persistent symptoms, mental and physical, some of which are fatigue, confusion, forgetfulness, rashes, and fevers.

AIDS

AIDS cases reported in the first 3 months of 1993 increased 21 percent over the same period the previous year.
—Centers for Disease Control, Atlanta, 1993

AIDS was the 15th cause of death in the United States in 1987, the 11th cause of death in 1989, and the 9th cause of death in 1992.
—National Center for Health Statistics, 1993

Predicted worldwide total infection with AIDS by the year 2000 will be 30 to 40 million.
—World Health Organization, 1993

The number of reported cases of AIDS worldwide as of January 1993 was 600,000 but estimates are that the real total is likely four times as high. Approximately 13 million people had become infected with HIV.
—World Health Organization, 1993

Twenty million deaths from AIDS are predicted by the year 2000.
—*AIDS in the World: Global Report*
Harvard University Press, 1992

AIDS is defined by the Centers for Disease Control as of July 1993 as "a specific group of diseases or conditions which are indicative of severe immuno suppression related to infection with the human immunodeficiency virus (HIV)." Extensive research and expenditure of money has not resulted in a cure for AIDS. There has been confirmation that the free radical is a factor in the initiation of AIDS and several papers on this topic were presented at the conference on "AIDS, HIV Infection and Free Radical" that took place in Les Deux Alpes, France, in January 1993. The National Institutes of Health announced at a conference on November 10, 1993, that studies indicate HIV blocks the body's defense against free radicals. Dr. Howard Greenspan, chairman of the conference, said that the abundance of free radicals amplifies the destructive effect of the virus.

▲

"Health becomes the freedom not to react to things, but to respond and have many different options—not to be trapped by an old belief about life."
—BILL MOYERS, *Healing and the Mind*, 1993

▲

AGING

The first research with free radicals and human health, done in the 1950s, was focused on their relation to aging. Many hundreds of medical articles since then confirm that aging is fundamentally a manifestation of free radical damage to the body cells. This results in a gradual reduction of health—the symptoms we refer to as aging.

Cross-linking, the fusion of side-by-side molecules, is often caused by free radicals. Free radicals cause bonding between molecules in the collagen and elastin, corrective tissue found in tendons, cartilage, and in skin. This results in wrinkles and the loss of flexibility associated with aging.

The overall effect of free radicals is to weaken cells and limit their ability to perform their function. This is described as aging. Researchers have found that workers at nuclear power plants age at a much faster rate, and the researchers' conclusion is that the constant exposure to radiation increases the workers' rate of aging.

These are only the most prevalent conditions linked to free radical damage. Free radicals have also been connected with numerous other diseases, including influenza, kidney and liver problems, Parkinson's disease, pancreatitis, and digestive diseases.

▲

"It isn't that they can't see the solution, they
can't see the problem."
—G. K. Chesterton

▲

Now that we have discussed the problem, the six chapters in Part II will present six avenues to pursue for some solutions.

RESOURCES

The following is a list of medical journal articles relating free radicals with cancer, heart disease, arthritis, mental disorders, cataracts, asthma, multiple sclerosis, tuberculosis, chronic fatigue syndrome, candidiasis, AIDS, and aging. This is followed by a resource section on how to obtain these articles.

Cancer
"Major Alterations in the Nucleotide Structure of DNA in Cancer of the Female Breast"
Donald Malins and Russom Haimanot
Cancer Research 51:5430–32, Oct. 1, 1991

Deadly Deceit
J. Gould and B. Goldman
Four Walls Eight Windows, 1991

"The Role of Oxygen Radicals as a Possible Mechanism of Tumor Promotion"
W. Troll
Annual Review of Pharmacol Toxicol 25:509–28, 1985

"Increasing Metastic Potential Is Associated with Increasing Genetic Inability of Clones Isolated from Murine Neoplasms"
M.A. Cifone
Proceedings of the National Academy of Science 78:6949–52

"Mutations in the p53 Gene in Primary Breast Cancers"
R.J. Osborne et al.
Cancer Research 512:6194–98, Nov. 15, 1991

"Evidence Implicating at Least Two Genes on Chromosome 17p in Breast Carcinogens"
C. Coles et al.
Lancet 336:761–63, 1990

"Severe Impairment of Antioxidant System in Human Hepatoma"
G.C. Guidi
Cancer 58:1658–62, Oct. 15, 1986

"Superoxide Dismutase Glutathione and Catalase in the Red Cells of Patients with Malignant Lymphoma"
M. Bewick et al.
British Journal of Haematology 65:347–50, March 1987

"Superoxide Dismutase Activity in Leukemia Blasts of Children with Acute Leukemia"
K. Yoshimitsu
Acta Paediatr Scand 73:92–196, Jan. 1984

"Cell Differentiation, Aging and Cancer"
L.W. Oberley et al.
Med Hypothesis 61:249–68, March 1980

"Cancer and Free Radicals"
W.A. Pryor
In *Antimutagenesis and Anticarcinogenesis Mechanisms,*
ed. D. Shankel, Plenum Press, 1986, pp. 45–49.

"Free Radicals in Tumor Protection"
T.W. Kensler
Advances in Free Radical Biology and Medicine
2:347–87, 1986

Heart Disease

"Oxygen Free Radicals and Heart Failure"
K. Prasad
Angiology 39:417–20, May 1988

"Evidence of Direct Toxic Effects of Free Radicals on
Myocardium"
K.P. Burton
Free Radical Biol Med 4:15–24, 1988

"Evaluation of Free Radical Injury to Myocardium"
K.A. Reimer
Toxicol Pathol 18:470–80, 1990

"Oxygen Radicals and Atherosclerosis"
K. Carpenter et al.
Klin Wochenschr 59:1039–45, 1991
This article discusses how free radicals may cause lesions
in the arteries. It is available from Dr. K. Carpenter,
Dept. of Pathology, University of Cambridge, Cambridge
CB21QP, England.

Arthritis

"Oxygen Radicals, Inflammation and Arthritis"
R.A. Greenwald
Seminar Arthritis and Rheumatism 20:219–40, Feb. 1991

"Anti-Radical Enzymes Oxygenated Free Radicals and
Peroxidation in Rheumatoid Polyarthritis"
A. Abella et al.
Revue Rheumatism 57:855–61, Dec. 1990

"Inhibitory Action of Tiopronin on Free Radicals"
M. Ronmain et al.
Revue Rheumatism 56:34–37, April 30, 1989

"Treatment of Inflammatory Arthritis with Oxygen Radical
Scavengers"
R.A. Greenwald
Journal of Free Radical Biological Medicine 2:367–68,
1986

"Free Radicals and Anti-Inflammatory Drugs"
H. Vapaatalo
Medical Biology 64:1–7, 1986

Diabetes

"Free Radicals and Diabetes"
L.W. Oberley
Journal of Free Radical Biological Medicine 5:113–24,
1988

"Involvement of O_2 Radicals in 'Autoimmune' Diabetes"
I.N. Nomikos
Immun Cell Biol 67:85–87, Feb. 1989

"Alterations in Free Radical Tissue Defense Mechanisms in Streptozocin-Induced Diabetes in Rats"
S.A. Wohaieb
Diabetes 36:1014–18, Sept. 1987

Mental Disorders

"Oxygen Radicals and Neuropsychiatric Illness"
J.B. Lohr
Archives of General Psychiatry 48:1097–1104, 1991

"Free Radical Theory of Aging: A Hypothesis on Pathogenesis of Senile Dementia of the Alzheimer's Type"
D. Harman
Journal of the American Aging Association 16:23–30, 1993

"The Risk Factors for Alzheimer's Disease: A Review and a Hypothesis"
A.S. Henderson
Acta Psychiatric Scandinavia 78(3):257–75, Sept. 1988

"Involvement of Free Radicals in Dementia of the Alzheimer Type"
L. Volicer and P.B. Crino
Neurobiological Aging 11:567–71, Sept.–Oct. 1990

"Reversal of Age-Related Increase in Brain Protein Oxidation, Decrease in Enzyme Activity and Loss in Temporal and Spatial Memory by Chronic Administration of the Spintrapping Compound N-tert-butyl-alpha-phenylnitone"
J.M. Carnery
Proceedings of the National Academy of Science 88:3633–36, May 1, 1991

"Fallout and the Decline of Scholastic Aptitude Scores"
E.J. Sternglass and S. Bell
Paper presented at the Annual Meeting of the American
Psychological Association, NYC, Sept. 3, 1979

"Oxidation-Reduction and the Brain"
A. Hoffer
J. Orthomol Psychiatry 12:292–301, 1983

"Free Radicals, Lipid Peroxidation and Parkinson's
Disease"
M.T. Smith, M.S. Sandy, and D. DiMonte
Lancet 1:38, 1987

"Increased Indices of Free Radical Activity in the
Cerebralspinal Fluid of Patients with Tardive Dyskinesia"
J.B. Lohr et al.
Biological Psychiatry 28:535–39, 1990

"Oxygen Free Radicals and Brain Dysfunction"
James Jesberger and Steven Richardson
International Journal of Neuroscience 57:1–17, 1991

Cataracts

"Micronutrients and Age-Related Cataracts"
R. Jacques and A. Taylor
In *Micronutrients in Health and Disease Prevention,* ed.
A. Bendich, New York, 1991, pp. 369–79

"India-U.S. Case Control Study of Age-Related Cataracts"
M. Mohan et al.
Archives of Ophthalmology, 1989, pp. 670–76

"A Possible Role for Vitamin C and E in Cataract
Prevention"
J.M. Robertson et al.
American Journal of Clinical Nutrition 12:183–46, 1993

"Increased Incidence of Cataracts and Lipid Peroxides"
K. Yagi
Clin Chem Acta 80:355–60, 1977

"Role of Oxygen Free Radicals in Retinal Damage
Associated with Experimental Uveitis"
N.A. Rao
Transactions of the American Opthalmological Society
88:797–850, 1990

"Free Radicals in Medicine: Involvement in Human
Disease"
P.A. Southern
Mayo Clinic Proceedings 63:390–408, 1988

Asthma
"The Role of Free Radicals in Airway Obstruction in
Asthmatic Patients"
Hiroshi Kanazawa et al.
Chest 100:1319–22, Nov. 1991

Multiple Sclerosis
"Increased Free Radicals in Multiple Sclerosis"
The Nutrition Report
10:70, 1992

"Evidence for Increased Lipid Peroxidation in Multiple
Sclerosis"
P. Toshniwal and E. Zarling
Neurochemical Research 17:205–7, 1992

Tuberculosis

"The Impact of Human Immunodeficiency Virus on Presentation and Diagnosis of Tuberculosis in a Cohort Study in Zambia"
A.M. Elliot et al.
Journal of Tropical Medical Hygiene 96:1–11, 1993

"Pleural Effusion, Tuberculosis and HIV-1 Infection in Kigali, Rwanda"
J. Batungwanayho et al.
AIDS 7(1):73–79, 1993

OTHER RELEVANT READING

Memoirs
  Andrei Sakharov
  Knopf, New York, NY, 1990

AIDS in the World: A Global Report
  ed. Jonathan Mann et al.
  Harvard University Press, 1992

Chronic Fatique Syndrome
"History of Chronic Fatigue Syndrome"
  S.E. Straus
  Review of Infectious Disease 13 (Suppl. 1) 2–7

"Immunologic Abnormalities in Chronic Fatigue
  Syndrome"
  Klimas et al.
  Journal of Clinical Microbiology, June 1990

"Chronic Fatigue Syndrome: Clinical Condition Associated Immune Activation"
Levy et al.
Lancet, Sept. 21, 1991

"A Chronic Illness Characterized by Fatigue, Neurologic and Immunologic Disorders and Active Human Herpesvirus Type 6 Infection"
Buchwald et al.
Annals of Internal Medicine, Jan. 15, 1992

"Lymphocyte Phenotype Function in Chronic Fatigue Syndrome"
Straus et al.
Journal of Clinical Immunology, Jan. 1993

Chronic Fatigue Syndrome: A Summary Study
National Institute of Allergy and Infectious Diseases, Feb. 1993

Environmental Illness
Human Ecology and susceptibility to the Chemical Environment
T.G. Randolph
Charles C. Thomas, Springfield, IL, 1962

E.I. Syndrome
Sherry Rogers, M.D.
Prestige Publishing, Syracuse, NY

Tired or Toxic?
Sherry Rogers, M.D.
Prestige Publishing, Syracuse, NY

Antioxidant Adaptation: Its Role in Free Radical Pathology
S. Levine and P. Kidd
Allergy Research Group, Biocurrents Division, 1986

Candidiasis

"Tissue Induced Candida Albicans: Mental and
Neurobiological Manifestations"
C.O. Truss
Journal of Orthomolecular Psychiatry 7:17–37, 1978

"The Role of Candida Albicans in Illness"
C.O. Truss
Journal of Orthomolecular Psychiatry 10:228–38, 1981

"Oral Candidiasis in High Risk Patients as the Initial
Manifestation of the Acquired Immunodeficiency
Syndrome"
R. Klein et al.
New England Journal of Medicine 311:354–58, Aug. 9,
1984

The Yeast Connection
W.C. Crook
Professional Books, Jackson, TN, 1984

AIDS

Papers presented at the Seminar on AIDS, HIV Infection
and Free Radicals, January 22–23, 1993, at Les Deux Alpes,
France:

"Presentation of the HIV Virus Structure and Replication"
J.C. Chermann

"Mechanisms of Gene Expression by the Nuclear Factor
NFKB"
P. Baeuerle

"Effects of UV Radiations on HIV Replication"
G. Poli

"Activation of HIV Virus by Oxygen Radicals"
J. Piette

"Ascorbate in HIV Infected Cells"
S. Harakeh

"Inhibition of HIV Replication by Cysteine Derivative"
W. Droge

"Acquired Immunodeficiency Without Evidence of Infection with Human Immunodeficiency Virus Types 1 and 2"
J. Laurence
Lancet 340:273–74, August 1, 1992

"Clue Is Reported to Speed of AIDS—HIV May Destroy Ability to Process Corrosive Type of Molecule, Studies Say"
New York Times, Nov. 14, 1993, p. A27

For a report on the incidence of AIDS:
The HIV/AIDS Surveillance Report
Division of HIV/AIDS
National Centers for Disease Control
Atlanta, GA 30333
(800) 458-5231
This free quarterly report lists the incidence of AIDS by category and geography.

Aging
"Free Radical Pathology in Age-Associated Disease"
E. Cranton and J. Frackelton
Journal of Holistic Medicine 6: Spring–Summer 1984

"Free Radicals and the Origin, Evolution and Present Status of the Free Radical Theory of Aging"
Denham Harman
In *Free Radicals in Molecular Biology Aging and Disease*, New York, Raven, 1984

"Free Radicals in Biological Systems"
W.A. Pryor
Journal of Gerontology 35:45–46, 1980

"Cross-Linking of Collagen in the Presence of Oxidizing Lipid"
F. Sundholm
Lipids 13:755–57, 1978

"Antioxidants and Aging"
R.G. Cutler
American Journal of Clinical Nutrition 53:373S–379S, 1991

Longevity
J. Bjorksten
Bjorksten Research Foundation, 1981, P.O. Box 9444, Madison, WI 53715

"Radiation Exposure and Human Species Survival"
R. Bertell
Environmental Health Review, June 1981, pp. 43–55

Other Diseases

"Oxygen Radicals in Influenza Induced Pathogenesis and Treatment with Pyran Polymer-Conjugated SOD"
T. Oda et al.
Science 224:974–76, May 26, 1989

"Oxygen Free Radicals in Nephrology"
C. Canavese et al.
International Journal of Artificial Organs 10:379–89,
Nov. 1987

"Oxygen Derived Free Radicals Promote Hepatic Injury in
the Rat"
M.J. Arthur
"Gastroenterology" 89:1114–24, Nov. 1985

"Oxygen Radicals"
A.M. Michelson
Agents Actions Supplement 11:179–201, 1982

"Environment, Genetics and Parkinson's Disease"
J. Poirier et al.
Canadian Journal of Neurological Science 18:70–76,
Feb. 1991

"Free Radicals in Digestive Diseases"
T. Yoshikawa
Nippon Ronen Igakkai Zasshi 27:155–60, March 1990

"Role of Oxygen Derived Free Radicals in the Pathogenesis
of Gastric Mucosal Lesions in Rats"
T. Yoshikawa
Journal of Clinical Gastroenterology 12:65–71, 1990

RESOURCES FOR PART I

To Obtain Copies of Medical Journal Articles

There are more than 3,000 orthodox biomedical and health journals regularly published. The National Library of Medicine places abstracts of every article from every journal on computer databases and this is available to everyone. The information contains the latest in conventional treatments and discussions of diseases. Also in the database is every article on prevention, nutrition, and dietary supplements found in mainstream medical journals. Seven regional libraries located at major medical colleges can help you with a search or article request. Many public libraries have access to MEDLARS databases and can perform searches for a cost of between $10 and $50.

For More Information:
MEDLARS
   National Library of Medicine
   8600 Rockville Place
   Bethesda, MD 20894
   (800) 638-8480
   FAX (301) 496-0822

Another Source for a Computer Readout Is:
Life Services
   MEDLARS Service
   (800) 542-3230
   Prices are from $20 to $40

Those who are interested in reading any of the articles listed in this book may go in person to:
New York Academy of Medicine
2 East 103rd Street
New York, NY 10029
(212) 876-8200
FAX (212) 722-7650
Or you may order copies of articles by mail from them for a fee of $8 per article prepaid. The volume, date, and page numbers should be included. Orders are processed within five days. For quicker service, articles may be faxed the next day for a fee of $16 per article.

Further Reading on Free Radicals
"The Possible Role of Free Radical Reactions in
   Carcinogenesis"
   H.B. Demopoulos et al.
   Journal of Environmental Pathology and Toxicology,
   1980, pp. 272–303

"The Development of Secondary Pathology with Free
   Radicals: Reactions as a Threshold Mechanism"
   H.B. Demopoulos et al.
   Journal of American Col Toxicol, 1983, pp. 173–84

"Oxygen Free Radicals Linked to Many Diseases"
   J.L. Marx
   Science, Jan. 30, 1987, pp. 249–531

"Natural Chemicals Now Called Major Cause of Disease"
   Jane Brody
   New York Times, April 26, 1988

"Free Radical"
   Natalie Angier
   New York Times Magazine, April 25, 1993, p. 62

"Free Radicals, Anti-Oxidants and Human Disease"
   B. Halliwell
   Journal of Laboratory and Clinical Medicine
   119(6):598–620, June 1992

"Oxygen Derived Free Radicals in Postischemic Tissue
   Injury"
   J.M. McCord
   New England Journal of Medicine 312:159, 1985

"Role of Free Radicals in Mutation, Cancer, Aging and the
   Maintenance of Life"
   Denham Harman
   Radiation Research 16:753–54, 1962

"Free Radical Theory of Aging"
   Denham Harman
   Journal of Gerontology, Oct. 23, 1968

"Free Radicals in Biological Systems"
W.A. Pryor
Scientific American, August 1970

"Free Radicals in Medicine: Involvement in Human Disease," Parts I and II
P.A. Southern and G. Powis
Mayo Clinic Proceedings 63:390–408, 1988

"Oxygen Derived Free Radicals: Pathophysiology and Implications"
Mark Hitt, DVM
Compendium Small Animal, Vol. 10, 1988, 8:939–46

"Free Radical Biology: Xenobiotics, Cancer and Aging"
W.A. Pryor
New York Academy of Sciences Annals, Vol. 393, 1982, pp. 1–22

"Oxygen Poisoning and X-irradiation: A Mechanism in Common"
R. Gerschman et al.
Science 119:623, 1954

"Oxygen and Oxy-Radicals in Chemistry and Biology"
M. Rogers and E. Powers
New York, Academic Press, 1981

"Life Extension"
Durk Pearson and Sandy Shaw
Warner Books, 1982
The first popular book on the subject of free radicals and how they affect health, aging in particular.

PART II

SIX WAYS TO COUNTERACT FREE RADICALS

"In the middle of difficulty lies opportunity."
—*Albert Einstein*

▲

"Although free radicals are ubiquitous, they are by no means omnipotent."
—BRIAN LIEBOVITZ, Ph.D., "Aspects of Free Radical Reactions in Biological Systems: Aging," *Journal of Gerontology*, 1980, Vol. 35

▲

HOW TO IMPROVE YOUR BODY'S DEFENSES AGAINST EXCESS FREE RADICALS

In 1968, researchers found that the body makes an enzyme that counters free radicals and keeps them in check. These enzymes stop free radical chain reactions before they are out of control. This discovery opened the door to understanding that we are not totally vulnerable to free radical damage; there is something we can do to compensate by augmenting these enzymes along with the nutrients that are now known to counter free radicals: the antioxidants. The first two chapters in Part II discuss food and nutritional supplements necessary to maintain this balance. Once you know the controllable variables that determine the rate of free radical reactions discussed in the next four chapters of Part II you can utilize them to make substantial improvements in your health. In addition to good nutrition and dietary supplements, these variables are exercise, stress reduction, exposure to full-spectrum light, and pollution avoidance. The use of protective foods, which remove radical-forming toxins, and specific scavenging supplements are sure ways to counter free radicals. Exercise and mental attitude create chemicals called endorphins that enhance the immune system and bolster it to resist being overwhelmed by free radicals (see chapters 5 and 6). Full-spectrum light feeds the pineal gland, which in turn fortifies immunity to counter excess free radicals. And of course, last but not least, it is essential to avoid pollution as much as possible. Chapter 8 points out poisons you might not have thought of and gives pointers for avoiding them.

The recipes in Part III, which are gathered together in complete menus, show you how to make a meal utilizing the protective foods, so that the information on food in Chapter 3 is immediately useful because it can be translated into dinner with the guidance of a complete menu.

Once you have gathered what you need from these chapters, the practical leads in the section on resources in Part IV will be an invaluable guide to help you to incorporate changes based on what you think is the most relevant for you.

CHAPTER 3

Food—The Delicious Fortifier

"Let food be your medicine, and medicine be your
food."   —*Hippocrates*

*T*he best foods for fighting free radicals are whole, natural,
traditional foods—the Paleolithic menu of grains, vegetables,
and beans with some sea vegetables, nuts and seeds and
sprouts. These foods contain what are referred to as free radical
scavengers, or antioxidants, which can hold in check the excess
aberrant molecules formed from exposure to pollutants and to
stress. They both detoxify and nutrify, and when they are
prepared well, as shown in the tasty complete menus and
recipes in Part III, they appeal to the most sophisticated food
critic.

This eating plan is consistent with the medical establish-
ment's recommendations. It is also optimum for a stronger
immunity, increased vitality, and healthier "no-diet" weight
loss. This is the way to tap into your own Fountain of Youth.

▲

"God in His infinite wisdom neglected
nothing, and if we would eat our food without

trying to improve, change or refine it, thereby
destroying its life-giving elements, it would
meet all the requirements of the body.''
—JETHRO KLOSS, *Back to Eden*, 1981

▲

It is no news that we are surrounded with unprecedented
levels of toxins: industrial poisons, chemical fertilizers, pesticides, and radiation are in our water, soil, food, and air. Even
small amounts of toxins do us harm by causing the accelerated
formation of free radicals. Government-declared permissible
levels of pollutants still cause health damage and early aging.
Is there anything to do about this? In addition to working for
societal change, the answer is that how much of an impact all
this has on you and your family is, to a large extent, determined
by *you*, because you control what you eat. Choose foods that
are low on the food chain to avoid toxins. And choose foods
with protective and healing powers.

AVOID TOXINS BY EATING FOODS
LOW ON THE FOOD CHAIN

The food chain starts with the smallest organisms—which
feed on the sun's energy, and are in turn eaten by progressively
larger organisms: grass grows, cows eat grass, humans eat
cows. Foods high on the food chain contain the most concentrated levels of toxic substances because the toxins become
more concentrated at each stage of the food chain.

▲

''Meats, animal protein, butter, cheese, fish,
animal fat, and all animal products are
completely unnecessary for maintaining your
health; these products as well as all other

manufactured and modern industrial products, may be abolished completely from your daily diet in order to reestablish and fortify your adaptability, imagination and judgment."
—George Ohsawa, *The Art of Peace*, 1952

▲

For example, a toxic chemical such as mercury, which causes free radical formation, may be released from a paper factory into a lake and be absorbed by algae, plankton, and bottom sediments. It may then be eaten by small fish, which are eaten by larger fish, increasing the concentration of mercury. These fish may swim down the river into the ocean, to be eaten by even larger fish, such as swordfish or tuna. In this way the large fish, which is high on the food chain, would contain a much greater concentration of mercury than originally in the algae in the lake where the toxin was released. You are not getting as healthy a lunch as you might think when you open a can of tuna!

So think low on the food chain to maximize the health benefits of the foods you eat. Center your diet on vegetables, grains, legumes, and fruits. Avoid foods high on the food chain, including meat, eggs, and dairy products—all from animals.

A book on the relation of humans to free-radical-causing radiation in the environment, *Strontium Metabolism in Man* (Academic Press, 1967), reported: "Milk and dairy products are the main source of dietary strontium-90 in the U.S." Which isn't surprising, because those foods are high on the food chain. A study on ducks around the Hanford, Washington, nuclear installation produced similar results. It found the concentration of cesium-137, which is emitted routinely from all nuclear plants, to be about 2,000 times the concentration in the ducks as in the original amount released.

▲

"I have no doubt that it is a part of the destiny
of the human race, in its gradual improvement,
to leave off eating animals."
—HENRY DAVID THOREAU

▲

A person who eliminates meat and dairy products from
his diet reduces his chance of heart attack by 90 percent,
according to a study by the vegetarian Seventh Day Adventists
published in 1975.

Besides aiding your health there are other benefits to
avoiding a meat-based diet, as clarified in *Diet for a New
America* by John Robbins (Stillpoint, 1987). This landmark
book on the many damages of a meat-based diet sums it up
this way: "If we kicked the meat habit there would be no need
for nuclear power plants. Our dependence on foreign oil would
be greatly reduced. We would have the time and resources to
develop solar and other environmentally sound energy
sources." That's because in addition to being ethically untena-
ble from the point of view of the environment and animal
rights, beef is an inefficient food. It takes six pounds of grain
to increase a steer's weight by one pound. If humans ate grain
instead of beef we'd have six times as much food available.
And meat production is extremely damaging to the environment. According to Robbins, stopping livestock production in
the United States would conserve 85 percent of the topsoil loss
and 50 percent of the water consumed for all purposes. The
beef industry is responsible for the loss of a quarter of the rain
forests in Central America and a loss of 40 percent of the
forests in Brazil since 1960.

▲

"The top nine sources of calories in the
American diet: whole milk, margarine, white

bread, rolls, sugar, 2% milk, ground beef,
wheat flour, pasteurized process American
cheese.''
—U.S. Department of Agriculture, 1992

▲

DEVELOP YOUR RESISTANCE TO TOXINS BY EATING TRADITIONAL FOODS

Up until about two centuries ago humans ate whole foods—namely grains, beans, and vegetables with a variety of wild game (which was not contaminated with modern toxins) and various condiments. It is this eating pattern that is suggested for optimum health in our toxic world. By avoiding the toxin-containing foods high on the food chain, this way of eating emphasizes the antioxidant nutrients and complete vegetarian proteins, calcium, minerals, and trace minerals.

If we assume that modern humans emerged about 30,000 to 50,000 years ago, then they have lived more than 95 percent of that time on high fiber, low fat, antioxidant-rich whole foods. It was only about 200 years ago that many dietary changes came about. With the Industrial Revolution, the intake of fat and sugar increased, while complex carbohydrates and antioxidant nutrients decreased. Since World War II we have witnessed a great increase in depleted, refined, and fractional foods, taking us yet further away from humans' traditional way of eating.

Researchers in Australia observed a group of aboriginal people who were extremely physically fit. After these energetic aboriginals were Westernized with low physical activity, a high intake of low-nutrient foods, high animal fat and low vegetable fiber, they manifested chronic diseases, including obesity, hypertension, high blood pressure, diabetes, and heart disease.

▲

"Some researchers estimate that dietary measures that control oxygen radical damage could give the average American five or more added years of healthy, productive life."
—JANE BRODY, "Natural Chemicals Now Called Major Cause of Disease," *The New York Times,* April 26, 1988

▲

America ranks eleventh in life expectancy in 1991 following Japan, Iceland, Sweden, Switzerland, Australia, the Netherlands, Canada, France, Norway, and Germany, according to the Metropolitan Life Insurance Company (*Statistical Bulletin,* Vol. 73, No. 3, July 1992). What makes Japanese people live the longest? It is noteworthy that in Japan the diet is very often vegetarian and as a result is full of antioxidants. And since their diet does not include dairy foods, they avoid the accumulated free-radical-causing toxins in milk and cheese. Also noteworthy is that Japanese national statistical longevity is achieved by tacking on about four years at life's upper end, not by a low infant mortality rate.

▲

"The cure of the part should not be attempted without treatment of the whole."
—PLATO, *The Republic*

▲

The grain-centered approach to eating, which is integral to all traditional cultures, provides fewer calories, less fat and sugar; and more fiber, nondairy calcium, and potassium. It also provides vitamin and mineral nutrients necessary to maintain good health in a toxic world.

ANTIOXIDANTS

The body's first line of protection against excess free radicals is in the internally generated antioxidant enzymes, which work to control the primary formation of free radicals. The prevention of the continuing proliferation of free radicals is carried out by the antioxidant nutrients, chiefly vitamins E and C and beta-carotene, along with the co-factors of the B vitamins, selenium, zinc, bioflavinoids, and many other factors found in plant foods. Minerals that fortify the antioxidant enzymes are selenium, copper, manganese, and zinc. These protective constituents in foods work together to block the further formation of free radicals. The antioxidants do this by donating an electron to stabilize the free radical, and in this way stop the domino effect that occurs when the free radical takes an electron from another molecule.

▲

"The underlying basis of Natural Hygiene is that the body is self-cleaning, self-healing, and self-maintaining. It is based on the idea that all the healing power of the universe is within the human body. We experience problems of ill health only when we break the natural laws of life."
—HARVEY AND MARILYN DIAMOND,
Fit for Life

▲

Both of these types of antioxidants have been shown to have a vital role in disease prevention. Many studies over the last twenty years attest to the protective effect of the antioxidant vitamins A, C, and E, and the antioxidant enzymes. Unfortunately, a large part of the population has inadequate intake of these protective nutrients which the modern diet, containing so much meat, fast food, and refined foods, is lacking.

▲

"The positive benefits of vegetables are many. In the course of metabolizing energy, the body's cells constantly generate hazardous molecules called free radicals, which can mutate genes and set the foundation for cancer. Most of the radicals are sopped up by the body's native antioxidant enzymes, but yellow and green vegetables contain a wealth of antioxidant compounds, including vitamins C and E and beta-carotene, the precursor to vitamin A."
—NATALIE ANGIER, "Chemists Learn Why Vegetables Are Good for You," *The New York Times*, April 13, 1993

▲

These three antioxidant vitamins—A, C, and E—stabilize free radicals by donating an electron. And they work together to back each other up—teamwork makes them each most effective. Once they have donated an electron they need it to be replaced, so vitamin C might support vitamin E's effectiveness by handing it an electron, once it has given one away to quench a free radical. The eating plan in Part III provides a variety of these nutrients, which is more effective than consuming any of the nutrients alone.

Beta-carotene, a precursor to vitamin A, is formed in the body by the liver. Beta-carotene also works on its own and has antioxidant functions and is effective at scavenging free radicals. Research has shown a relation between higher levels of beta-carotene and lower levels of tumors and cancers and other degenerative disease. Beta-carotene and vitamin A also serve to enhance immune function. They are found in all green and yellow vegetables.

▲

"If your philosophy doesn't grow corn, I don't
want to hear about it."
—Sun Bear

▲

Vitamin C is known to act synergistically with vitamin E in preventing free radical damage to lipids (fats) in the body, thus protecting cell membranes and nerve sheaths. It can have an effect on the DNA in the cell to prevent the destruction free radicals can cause. Vitamin C also works along with the glutathione peroxidase enzyme to stop free radical chain reactions.

Other benefits of vitamin C are that it protects the immune system and facilitates many body processes. Most importantly, it forms the collagen that keeps the body together. Vitamin C is found in most vegetables and fruits, including broccoli, green peppers, leafy greens, and citrus fruits.

Vitamin E is an efficient scavenger of free radicals, and it is key to counteracting free radicals so they do not tear apart the cell membrane. It also prevents platelets in the arteries from clumping together and blocking the free flow of blood, which can often result in stroke or heart disease. It defends the DNA in cells, thus possibly avoiding cancerous mutations. It is believed to have anticarcinogenic properties. Vitamin E is found in whole grains, nuts, and cold-pressed oils.

▲

"If I had to recommend one nutrient above
any other to include in a person's low-fat,
high-fiber diet to reduce the risk of disease, it
would have to be beta carotene. Beta carotene

is the most potent free radical neutralizer known today.''
—CHARLES SIMON, M.D., *Cancer and Nutrition*, 1983

▲

ANTIOXIDANTS AND FOOD SOURCES

Nutrient: Beta-carotene—Vitamin A

FOOD SOURCE	AMOUNT PER SERVING (100 grams/3½ ounces)
Vegetables:	
carrots	11,000 IU
leafy greens	7,000 to 10,000 IU
squash	7,000 IU
broccoli	3,300 IU
Beans:	
chick peas	50 IU
soybeans	30 IU
Sea vegetables:	
nori	20,000 IU
hijiki	150 IU
wakame	140 IU
Fruit:	
cantaloupe	3,400 IU
apricots	2,700 IU
peaches	1,330 IU
watermelon	590 IU
apples	117 IU

Suggested Daily Intake:
2 leafy green vegetables
2 yellow vegetables

RDA (Recommended Daily Allowances):
5000 IU or 3 mg of beta-carotene

Protective: Additional supplements not necessary if food intake is adequate.

Nutrient: Vitamin C

Food Source	Amount per Serving (100 grams/3½ ounces)
Vegetables:	
leafy greens	150 mg
broccoli	113 mg
brussels sprouts	100 mg
cauliflower	78 mg
cabbage	47 mg
Fruit:	
strawberries	59 mg
oranges	50 mg
cantaloupe	33 mg
nectarines	13 mg
apricots	10 mg

Suggested Daily Intake:
3 vegetables
1 fruit in season

RDA:

60 mg

Protective:

Additional supplements may be used depending on stress and pollution (see following chapter).

"Remedies from chemicals will never stand in favorable comparison with the products of nature—the living cell of the plant, the final result of the rays of the sun."
—THOMAS EDISON

Nutrient: Vitamin E

FOOD SOURCE	AMOUNT PER SERVING (100 grams/3½ ounces)
Grains:	
oatmeal	3 to 4 IU
all whole grains	3 to 4 IU
Vegetables:	
leafy greens	1 to 4 IU
turnips	1 to 4 IU
Beans:	
all beans	1 to 4 IU
Vegetable oils: all cold-pressed unrefined	12 to 20 IU per tablespoon

Suggested Daily Intake:
3 vegetables
3 grains
2 teaspoons oil

RDA:
30 IU

Protective:
Additional supplements may be considered (see following chapter).

B COMPLEX CO-FACTORS FOR ANTIOXIDANTS

The B vitamins act as co-factors for the A, C, and E; a sort of backup system. They are able to recycle antioxidants that have already donated an electron to neutralize a free radical, and by refilling their own quota they are enabled to continue their work of combating marauding free radicals.

SOME REASONS FOR DECREASED AVAILABILITY OF ANTIOXIDANT VITAMINS

Sometimes, even if you eat foods containing sufficient quantities of A, C, and E antioxidants, your body cannot make use of all the available nutrients. That happens for a variety of reasons, as the table on the next page summarizes.

NUTRIENT	REASONS FOR DECREASED AVAILABILITY
Vitamin A, beta-carotene	alcohol consumption pollution lack of zinc chemicalized foods
Vitamin C	stress use of drugs and alcohol aspirin smoking air pollution fluoride in water infection
Vitamin E	birth control pills rancid fats chloride
B complex	stress refined foods overcooked vegetables

▲

"Cauliflower is nothing but cabbage with a college education."
—MARK TWAIN

▲

OTHER ANTIOXIDANTS IN FOODS

Aside from these key and essential antioxidant vitamins there are other components in foods that have antioxidant capabilities. Some of these are:

COMPONENT	FOOD SOURCE
Allylic sulfides	garlic, onions
Catechins	green tea, berries
Bioflavinoids	most fruits and vegetables
Lycopene	tomatoes, red grapefruit
Monoterpenes	parsley, carrots, broccoli, cabbage, squash, yams, tomatoes, peppers, citrus fruits
Phenolic acids	parsley, carrots, broccoli, cabbage, whole grains, berries
Sulfur containing compounds cysteine, methionine, taurine	cabbage family vegetables, brussels sprouts, cauliflower, broccoli, kale, onions, watercress, mustard greens, chard
Protease inhibitors	the legume family: green peas, soybeans, lima beans, adzuki, pinto beans, kidney beans, split peas
Glutathione	carrots, spinach, tomatoes, apples
Phospholipids	nori sea vegetables

—Natalie Angier
"Chemists Learn Why Vegetables Are Good for You"
The New York Times, April 13, 1988
Sara Shannon, *Diet for the Atomic Age*

ENZYME ANTIOXIDANTS AND FOOD SOURCES FOR THEIR NUTRIENTS

The three main antioxidant enzymes produced by the body are superoxide dismutase, catalase, and glutathione peroxidase. They are fabricated out of the body's general nutrient bank with particular emphasis on a few minerals.

Nutrient: Selenium

FOOD SOURCE	AMOUNT PER SERVING (100 grams/3½ ounces)
Grains:	
brown rice	40 mcg
barley	30 to 40 mcg
pasta	0 to 40 mcg
oats	3 to 11 mcg
Vegetables:	
broccoli	amounts vary with soil
garlic	conditions
Fish:	
all fish	15 to 40 mcg

Suggested Daily Intake:
3 servings of grains

RDA:
50 to 200 mcg

Protective:

Selenium may be low in foods, especially nonorganic foods, due to depleted soil, so supplementation is suggested (see chapter 4).

Nutrient: Zinc

FOOD SOURCE	AMOUNT PER SERVING (100 grams/3½ ounces)
Grains:	
oatmeal	14 mg
corn	2.5 mg
brown rice	1.5 mg
Vegetables:	
green peas	1.6 mg
parsley	0.9 mg
cabbage	0.8 mg
carrots	0.5 mg
watercress	0.5 mg
Beans:	
split peas	4.2 mg
black beans	0.4 mg
lentils	0.2 mg
Nuts and seeds:	
pecans	4.5 mg
walnuts	3.6 mg
pumpkin seeds	2.6 mg

FOOD SOURCE	**AMOUNT PER SERVING** **(100 grams/3½ ounces)**
Fish:	
haddock	1.7 mg
shrimp	1.5 mg

Suggested Daily Intake:
Grains and vegetables and nuts

RDA:
15 mg

Protective: Often low in foods, especially nonorganic foods, due to depleted soil, so supplementation is suggested (see next chapter).

▲

"A smiling face is half the meal."
—LATVIAN PROVERB

▲

Sprouts contain SOD (superoxide dismutase), catalase, and other enzymes. Good sprouts are lentils, sunflower seeds, mung beans, and clover. See more about sprouts and how to grow your own at the end of Part III.

VEGETARIAN WHOLE FOODS ENHANCE IMMUNE FUNCTION

Whole foods are the best source of vitamin B_6 and zinc, which are necessary for a strong thymus gland. The thymus transforms white blood cells into T cells, whose job it is to kill foreign cells and cancer cells. The thymus also produces hormones that regulate the immune system.

NUTRIENT	FOOD SOURCE	REASONS FOR DECREASED AVAILABILITY
B_6	whole grains, beans, cabbage, nuts	not in refined foods; depleted by stress; destroyed by birth control pills, antibiotics, alcohol, high fat
Zinc	whole grains, green vegetables, seafood	soil depletion, food processing, depleted by stress, alcohol, excess copper (in water from pipes, or in a multisupplement)

In times of stress, or if your usual diet is low in these nutrients, it may be wise to assure availability of B_6 and zinc by taking a supplement.

VEGETABLES, GRAINS, AND BEANS PROVIDE POLLUTION PROTECTION

The whole-food, vegetarian way of eating provides protection from all pollutants to some degree. These foods, low on the food chain, contain lower concentrations of toxins for you to ingest. The following list give some toxins and their sources and the foods that are generally protective. For more details see my study of the subject in *Diet for the Atomic Age* (Avery, 1987).

POLLUTANT	SOURCE	PROTECTIVE FOODS

Lead	lead paint
	car exhaust
	pottery glaze
	tobacco smoke
	newsprint
	hair dye
		cabbage family vegetables
		sea vegetables
		leafy green vegetables
		  (for their calcium
		  content—calcium
		  displaces lead)
		whole grains
		beans

Cadmium	tobacco smoke
	fertilizer
		cabbage family vegetables
		sea vegetables
		green vegetables (for their
		  zinc content—zinc
		  displaces cadmium)
		whole grains
		beans

Fluoride	tap water toothpaste	cabbage family vegetables sea vegetables
Mercury	chemical fertilizers dental amalgams (fillings) pesticides	cabbage family vegetables whole grains beans

Aluminum	water-base paint
	cooking utensils
	tap water
	aluminum foil
	antacids
		leafy green vegetables
		  (for their calcium
		  content)
		whole grains
		beans

BALANCE: THE IMPORTANCE OF
THE PROPER RATIO OF FOODS

A healthy vegetarian diet counters free radicals, fortifies the immune function, and protects from pollution. It helps maintain a neutral pH of the blood, neither too acid nor too alkaline. Meat proteins are acid, and on the other end of the spectrum, fruits and sweets are alkaline: too much of either can affect the pH and disrupt the optimum balance. Grains, beans, and vegetables are in the middle range of pH, so they produce a healthy balance between acid and alkaline. That balance provides the best transport medium for hormones to reach glands and organs, thereby helping to keep the body healthy overall. The way to maintain this mid-range body chemistry is generally to eat foods in a certain proportion to each other in each meal, with grains being 30 to 40 percent, vegetables 60 to 70 percent, and the balance made up of either a small serving of fish or a soybean product, sea vegetables, nuts, seeds, or a fruit. This was the traditional diet for human beings up until the Industrial Age, when we began to eat more meats and fats and oils. Note that the best ratio of grains to vegetables will vary from person to person and depends on the individual's constitution and condition at the time, what season it is, and other factors. So there is a flexible area between 25 and 50 percent grains that depends on these variables. What is important is to understand that the ratio of foods to each other is important.

▲

"The formulation of a problem is often more essential than its solution."
—ALBERT EINSTEIN

▲

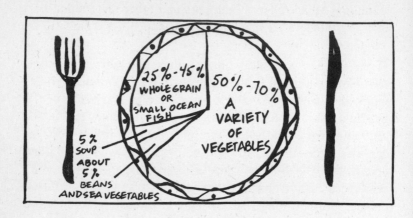

THE TRADITIONAL FOODS

Grains

Grains are important these days because they provide many important nutrients, while containing less toxins than foods from higher on the food chain. In the pioneering book that appeared in 1971, *Diet for a Small Planet*, Frances Moore Lappé introduced the idea to modern America that we *can* eliminate meat as a protein source and flourish with grains and beans and vegetables as most peoples had done for thousands of years. She built a convincing case for using grains as a staple as "a way for you to minimize the amount of ecologically concentrated pesticide and heavy metal you ingest, by eating low on the food chain."

Grains help to maintain the body's mid-range pH. Being just about between acid and alkaline, they serve to keep the body chemistry in that optimum middle range. Grains also contain a broad range of nutrients and other factors that have specific functions that resist toxic chemicals and radiation— phytates and fiber bind with toxins to eliminate them. The bulking factor of grains lessens intestinal transit time, thus hastening elimination of all toxins. Vitamin E and selenium found in grains are antioxidants that help to eliminate free radicals. The mineral content of grains, including calcium, iron, and zinc, is important, and their B vitamins act as antioxidant co-factors. Vitamin B_6, which is taken out of refined grains and not replaced, is indispensable for the thymus gland, where the T cells of the immune system are formed.

Nutrients Found in Grains

NUTRIENTS (FOUND IN ALL GRAINS)	BENEFITS YOU
Fiber	binds with and helps rid body of toxins
Phytates	binds with toxins
B complex	antioxidant co-factors, fortifies immune system and nervous system
B_6 and zinc	essential for production of T cells and immune system
Vitamin E	antioxidant, helps circulation
Selenium	antioxidant

NUTRIENTS (FOUND IN ALL GRAINS)	BENEFITS YOU
Calcium	builds bones, blocks absorption of some toxins
Magnesium	helps maintain pH balance— soothing to nervous system
Chromium	helps stabilize blood sugar

Vegetables

Like grains, vegetables are also low on the food chain and they support the healthy mid-range pH of the body chemistry. Vegetables are the key sources of the antioxidant vitamins A, C, and E. They also contain the supportive co-factors of the B complex vitamins and zinc. Green vegetables are a good non-dairy source of calcium. The cabbage family vegetables (often called cruciferous) contain two amino acids, cysteine and methionine, which are antioxidants.

It is recommended to have several vegetables at each meal. The following three categories of vegetables should be represented on your plate every day:

Cabbage family of vegetables
bok choy, kohlrabi, broccoli, mustard greens, brussels sprouts, radishes, cabbage, red cabbage, cauliflower, rutabagas, Chinese cabbage, turnips, collards, watercress, kale, chard, parsley

Yellow and green vegetables
carrots, Swiss chard, collards, squash, corn, watercress

Leafy green vegetables
kale, spinach

Nutrients Found in Vegetables

NUTRIENTS	FOUND IN THESE VEGETABLES	BENEFITS YOU
Vitamin A	carrots, corn, green beans, kale, all leafy greens, squash, zucchini	antioxidant, defends against infection, maintains skin
B complex	all vegetables	antioxidant co-factor, fortifies immune system and nervous system
B_6 and zinc	all leafy greens, green peas	essential for production of T cells and immune function
Vitamin C	all green vegetables	antioxidant, supports adrenal glands, general detoxifier
Vitamin E	all leafy greens	antioxidant, helps circulation
Calcium	all green vegetables	builds bones, blocks absorption of some toxins
Magnesium	all vegetables	maintains pH balance, soothing to nervous system

NUTRIENTS	FOUND IN THESE VEGETABLES	BENEFITS YOU
Sulfur	all cabbage family	helps repair free radical damage to DNA, resists radiation and toxins
Potassium	all vegetables	maintains pH balance
Fiber	all vegetables	binds with and helps rid body of toxins

Seaweeds

Sea vegetables, especially nori, contain phospholipids, which are antioxidants. Sea vegetables are full of minerals and trace elements that are uniquely nutritious and protective. They contain the nutrient iodine, which is essential to protect against the absorption of radioactive iodine found in fallout and emissions from nuclear power plants. The calcium content of sea vegetables is especially high, and this is important for those who avoid high-on-the-food-chain dairy products. Sea vegetables also contain magnesium, potassium, and zinc, important nutrients in the fight against free radicals.

Sodium alginate, which is also found in sea vegetables, is a dependable and powerful protector against toxic substances. A study way back in 1964 demonstrated that sea vegetables could reduce by 50 to 80 percent the amount of radioactive strontium absorbed by the intestine. Aside from this it can remove strontium that has already been absorbed. So this is an important contribution to the menu.

Sea Vegetables
hijiki, kombu, wakame, arame, dulse, nori

Nutrients Found in Sea Vegetables

NUTRIENT	BENEFITS YOU
Vitamin B_{12}	builds red blood cells, essential for nervous system
Chromium	helps stabilize blood sugar
Iodine	maintains thyroid, blocks uptake of radioactive iodine-131
Zinc	antioxidant co-factor, essential for immune system
Sodium alginate	binds with toxic substances and radiation
Phospholipids	antioxidants

▲

"Change takes place from the inside out."
—EDGAR MITCHELL, Apollo 14 astronaut, 1993

▲

Beans

The people of many traditional cultures ate grains and beans together. This made a perfect complement because the amino acid lysine, which is missing in grains and needed to make complete protein, is found in beans. The 1971 book *Diet for a Small Planet* brought out this fact and illustrated this grain-bean food combining with some wonderful recipes. Since then it has become clear that grains and beans do not need to be combined at the same meal, that there is a sort of "protein pool" from which the body draws protein as needed.

The bean family contains protease inhibitors, which are antioxidants and have protective powers against some toxins. Beans are also a source of the antioxidant vitamins A, C, and E and the B complex and zinc co-factors.

Beans

adzuki beans, split peas, lentils, kidney beans, chickpeas, lima beans, soybeans, pinto beans

▲

"Red beans and ricely yours."
—LOUIS ARMSTRONG (the way he signed his letters)

▲

Nutrients Found in Beans

NUTRIENTS	FOUND IN THESE BEANS	BENEFITS YOU
Vitamin A	most beans	antioxidant, defends against infection, maintains skin
B complex	most beans	antioxidant co-factor, fortifies immune system and nervous system
Vitamin B_{12}	tempeh, miso	build red blood cells, essential for nervous system
Calcium	most beans	builds bones, blocks absorption of some toxins

Nutrients	Found in These Beans	Benefits You
Potassium	all beans	maintains pH balance
Iron	all beans	builds red blood cells, blocks uptake of plutonium
Zinc	all beans	antioxidant co-factor essential for immune system
Fiber	all beans	binds with and rids body of toxins
Zybicolin	miso	binds with and rids body of radioactive toxic substances

▲

"It is wonderful. If we choose the right diet, what an extraordinary small quantity would suffice."
—Gandhi

▲

Miso

Miso is a fermented soy product. Its detoxifying powers are legendary. It was used effectively by some of the Japanese survivors of the Nagasaki atomic bombing in 1945. They ate no sugar at all, and had miso daily and remained healthy. Part of miso's protective power is due to the enzymes it contains. Another part is due to zybicolin, a binding agent with properties that attract and bind with toxic elements and radioactive elements. This keeps the body from absorbing these poisons and stops the formation of excess free radicals. Miso is also a vegetarian source of B_{12}, which otherwise is found primarily in animal foods.

Nutrients Found in Miso

NUTRIENT	BENEFITS YOU
B complex vitamins	antioxidant co-factor, fortifies immune system and nervous system
Vitamin B_{12}	builds red blood cells, essential for the nervous system
Enzymes	helps digestion
Zybicolin	eliminates toxins

Nuts and Seeds

Nuts and seeds are a compact food: they contain everything necessary to grow a flower, tree, or bush. They supply concentrated protein, almost as much as meat, but are preferable because they are low on the food chain. They also provide the B complex vitamins, the antioxidant vitamin E, and zinc. Nuts and seeds also contain pectin and phytates, which eliminate toxins and thus offset formation of free radicals.

Nuts
filberts, walnuts, Brazil nuts, pistachio nuts, pecans, almonds, cashews

Seeds
sesame seeds, pumpkin seeds, sunflower seeds

Sprouts

There are many plants that can be grown indoors and eaten as sprouts. The seed germinates when water is added, and with this process increases the plant's nutrient content enormously. For example, the B vitamins can increase over 500 percent in the process of going from seed to sprout. Or consider that there are 12 milligrams of iron in 100 grams of alfalfa sprouts, while in that much spinach there are only 2.6 milligrams.

Sprouts grow to fifty times their volume. Five tablespoons of alfalfa seeds (costing about 25 cents) will grow to one pound. You can store seeds thirty to sixty years. Part III contains clear instructions for sprouting.

Leafy Green Sprouts
alfalfa, buckwheat, sunflower, clover, cabbage, garlic

Sprouted Beans
garbanzo, green peas, soy, mung, adzuki, lentils

Sprouted Grains
wheat, rye, barley

▲

"It makes an enormous difference to the soil when you work it with love. Then you are channeling into the soil higher energy and imbuing it with God-power."
—*The Findhorn Garden*, by the Findhorn Community, 1976

▲

CHOOSE ORGANIC FOOD FOR FEWER TOXINS AND MORE NUTRIENTS

You may select excellent foods and eat them in a good ratio to each other, but if they grow in an area full of pesticides, insecticides, fungicides, and the other chemicals used in modern food production, your health could still be at risk. These polluted foods will not provide the necessary nutrients for abundant health. Chemicalized and depleted soil makes depleted food, which makes depleted people.

ORGANIC FOOD HAS MORE VITALITY

Aside from the tangible factor of the nutrients contained in foods, the life-force or energy of a food is of great importance. This would be partly determined by the freshness of the food, and primarily by how chemical-free it is. More natural, organic growing conditions with a more mineralized and nutrient rich soil will, obviously, affect the food it produces. Ideally, it would be wonderful if we could provide at least a part of our own food from our own garden. A next best choice is to seek out organic foods. These are becoming increasingly available.

Organic certification is done by thirty-three certification organizations in the United States. Some of the names of the largest are the Organic Crop Improvement Association, the National Organic Farmers Association, and the California Certified Organic Farmers. The fine points of certifying a food as organic vary among these groups but all of them stipulate a waiting period of at least three years since using chemical pesticides and fertilizers on the soil. Certain other requirements vary. Call any certification organization for a set of their standards. One group you may call is the Organic Crop Improvement Association at (513) 592-4983. The consumer should look for the words "certified organic" on the label or in the store, and the name of the organization that does the certification. If it does not say it is certified and by whom, then it is most likely not organic.

▲

"Millions of pounds of synthetic pesticides applied to crops in 1965: 335. Millions of pounds of synthetic pesticides applied to crops in 1989: 806."
—*Nutrition Action* Newsletter, 1992

▲

There are 600 pesticides registered with the U.S. Environmental Protection Agency (EPA) and 496 leave residues on food. In order to register a pesticide, the EPA must show that it does not cause "unreasonable effects" to human beings or the environment. There have been several admissions over the last decade that some of these pesticides may be carcinogenic.

In particular, the EPA announced in February 1993 that there are 35 carcinogenic pesticides in foods. Banned and toxic insecticides such as chlordane and heptachlor are made exclusively for export and may return to your table in imported vegetables and fruits. In 1989, 806 million pounds of synthetic pesticides were applied to crops—compared to 335 million pounds in 1965.

Experiments have found that foods that are grown organically result in foods that are nutritionally superior. In 1974, a German professor and director of the Federal Institute of Research on the Quality of Plant Production, Werner Schuphan, published his findings based on his twelve-year experiment on nutrients in organically grown foods.

Schuphan found higher contents of minerals, potassium, iron, magnesium, and calcium. Spinach grown in organically fertilized soil contained from 64 to 78 percent more ascorbic acid; lettuce contained 59 percent more ascorbic acid. Protein increased in spinach from 4 to 6 percent, and in carrots 21 to 25 percent. Some of the amino acids that are found to be protective against toxins were increased. And, Schuphan wrote, "We may come to the conclusion that organic manuring unequivocally favors sulfur-containing methionine, one of the most important amino acids."

ORGANIC FOOD DOES NOT POLLUTE

Organic farmers use substances and techniques that do not pollute. They aim to sustain the vitality of the soil and to avoid chemicals, which can run off into our water supply. They utilize natural fertilizers such as plant matter, rock powders, and seaweed. Instead of overusing the soil they practice crop rotation to avoid soil depletion. Insects and rodents are managed by natural predators such as geese, or "good bugs" that consume "bad bugs." A depleted soil attracts more insects, so avoiding soil depletion caused by chemical fertilizers and intensive farming methods takes care of a lot of the insect infestation. Botanical insecticides may also be used.

▲

"Sales of organic food in 1992 climbed 15% to $1.4 billion for the industry's fourth consecutive year of double-digit growth."
—*Spectrum* magazine, No. 33, November 1993

See Part IV for resources for organic food and for gardening suggestions and books. Also note how to buy a share in Community Supported Agriculture (CSA) by making a lump-sum payment before the growing season to a CSA farm, for which you receive in exchange a regular supply of fresh organically grown vegetables and fruits.

EASY WAY TO WEIGHT LOSS

The average number of pounds men and women surveyed in 1992 said they were trying to lose was thirty, according to the *American Journal of Public Health*. And this is at a time when growing distrust of weight loss regimes and calorie counting, together with feminism, have combined to launch the anti-diet movement. Eating according to the plan outlined here is consistent with this sensible move away from restrictive and obsessive dieting. It will allow weight to normalize and health to improve, which will, in turn, further normalize the weight.

Crash dieting is unproductive. Experiments with lab animals have shown that when they were fed a small amount of food for a week and then a normal amount of food, they added fatty tissue—more than what would have been expected had they just eaten normally. Most people who have tried to quickly lose five pounds and then return to their usual food intake can attest to this. And in fact, 95 percent of dieters regain the weight they lost.

The thyroid is the gland that regulates your rate of metabolism. When you eat less it produces less regulating hormones. When you eat an appropriate amount for your energy needs, it regulates appropriately. So restricting food is no guarantee of permanent weight loss.

The choice of foods makes all the difference in weight loss. A whole-grain, vegetarian eating plan is ideal for bringing you to your ideal weight. People who eat very little meat and dairy products have less body fat. Those who have a vegetarian diet receive a good variety of nutrients and adequate protein.

This good supply of nutrients also assures a feeling of having been nutrified and allays the food cravings that often result from inadequate nutrition. Whole grains and vegetables also provide appetite-satisfying fiber, which is bulky and discourages overeating, making it effortless to lose weight.

Nutritionist Nathan Pritikin said: ''Much maligned carbohydrates turn out to be not only the healthiest kinds of foods we eat, but also the kinds that keep people slim.'' Besides the selection of foods, the ratio of one food to another is as important for weight loss as it is for health. Even though brown rice is an excellent food, if it is eaten exclusively it won't encourage health or weight loss. A balance between the complex carbohydrates of grains and beans, and the foods of the vegetable family, is a key to weight loss; 25 to 45 percent grains and the balance a variety of vegetables will build health and normalize weight.

Keep in mind that it is also true that exercise is essential to maintaining your ideal weight, Exercise elevates the basal metabolism and burns stored fat. Read Chapter 5 for inspiration.

According to a 1983 report (*Recent Advances in Obesity Research*, by John Libbey, London, 1983) the prevalence of obesity in the United States has doubled since 1900. It is estimated that half of women and a fourth of men are dieting to lose weight at any one time (*Journal of American Medical Association*, 1991, pp. 2811–12). So the nonstressful weight loss eating plan that maintains a normal weight is a blessing.

▲

''The headquarters for the biological and spiritual transformation of humanity, including the recovery of natural immunity against AIDS and other degenerative and immune deficiency

diseases, is the kitchen in every home and the eating place in every community.''
—Michio Kushi (the father of balanced eating through macrobiotics), *One Peaceful World*, 1987

▲

BE EMPOWERED

Your regular day-to-day food intake *can* make a major difference in your power to resist and block absorption of poisons. It *can* provide the protective antioxidants. To understand this puts you in an empowered, rather than a vulnerable, position. It allows you to choose to optimize yourself and to place yourself in the category of people who are healthy enough and independent enough to take steps to change the damage done to our earth, and to lead others to a new way of living with respect for nature and all life.

PROPER RATIO OF DAILY INTAKE OF FOODS

Tack up this chart in some convenient place to remind yourself of the important foods to emphasize and the approximate quantity and ratio of each.

Food Source	Ratio	Daily Serving	Serving Size
Grains:	25–45%		
whole grains		2 or 3	½ cup
pasta			

FOOD SOURCE	RATIO	DAILY SERVING	SERVING SIZE
Vegetables:	50–70%		
cabbage family		2 or 3	½ cup
leafy greens		2 or 3	
yellow		1 or 2	
Beans:	5%		
various beans		2	2 tablespoons
tempeh, tofu, T.V.P. (Textured Vegetable Protein)			
Sea vegetables	less than 5%	1	¼ cup
Seeds and nuts	less than 5%	1	¼ cup
Ocean fish	less than 5%	a few times per week	5–6 ounces
Fruit	less than 5%	1 or less	½ cup
Sprouts	less than 5%	2	½ cup

The serving sizes are approximate. The main point is to keep the ratio in mind: the proportion of one food to another. You may vary the serving sizes to suit your energy needs.

It is easy to see that a low-on-the-food-chain grain and vegetable diet, rich in antioxidants and substances needed by the antioxidant enzymes, is the most effective in promoting an optimum state of health. Thoughtful attention to your food will counter free radicals. Go on to the next chapter for the insurance policy of the judicious use of supplements, which may be necessary in our polluted and stressed era that generates excess free radicals.

Chapter 4

Supplements— The Equalizers

"An ounce of prevention is worth a pound of cure."   *—Old adage*

*B*ecause we are all living in a contaminated soup of pollutants, it is worthwhile exploring ways to lower our health risk. We can control our exposure to toxins to some extent by avoiding tap water, or by moving away from a particular toxic dump, for example. We may also counteract pollutants with a high-nutrient vegetarian eating plan. Yet with the extreme amounts of toxins that some of us are now exposed to, and may be in the future, it is worth exploring the protective and youth-extending use of supplements. It is important to note that counteracting toxins is not a cure. The cure is in eliminating these man-made poisons.

THE NEED FOR SUPPLEMENTS VARIES

There is a great variety of degrees of health within groups of people who are considered generally well. And in any one individual there is a potential for varying levels of health as well. There may be people who, due to their physical constitution and condition, can tolerate exposure to toxins much better than another person is able to. This ability was referred to by Dr. Roger Williams in the 1960s in his book *Biochemical Individuality*, in which he explains that everyone functions in a highly individualized way.

So there are no absolute amounts of foods or supplements that are appropriate for everyone. This chapter offers a guideline for meeting the demands of our extraordinarily stressful environment. It is based on the current research on free radicals and antioxidants, which has substantiated the body's ability, when well nutrified, to counteract the health damage of toxins and maintain a state of youthfulness as long as possible.

NUTRIENT SUPPLEMENTS MAY ENCOURAGE OPTIMUM HEALTH

Although they may be adequate to prevent deficiency diseases, the allowances of nutrients as suggested by the Food and Nutrition Board's Recommended Daily Allowances may be inadequate for people to maintain optimum health in our toxic world. Aside from this, the diet of many Americans is chronically under even these modest recommendations. The most recent survey, the Nationwide Food Consumption Survey (1987–1988), found the typical American diet provides less than the RDA for vitamins E and B_6, calcium, iron, magnesium, and zinc.

Given the fact that most of our diets are inadequate, that chemicalized soil produces depleted foods, and that high levels of environmental toxins *must* be countered by a nutrifying food intake in order to maintain and promote optimum health, fortification with supplements to some degree does make sense.

▲

"Every day, each cell in the body generates
tens of thousands of free radicals, by-products
of normal metabolism. They tend to undermine
neighboring molecules. Pollutants augment the
process. Antioxidants, which can neutralize
free radicals, are among the body's
mechanisms for stemming the damage."
—"Free Radical," NATALIE ANGIER, *The New
York Times*, April 25, 1993

▲

Supplements are in no way intended to make up for a fractionated factory food intake. They are meant to enhance a good eating plan, to fill in where foods may be lacking, and to augment when extra protection may be needed.

The most serious problem nowadays is that there is a grave imbalance: there are too many free radicals, and too few free radical fighters to offset them. Our body was designed to keep radicals in check and in the past, even when there were variations in the amounts of foods consumed, the level of stress, and the exposure to toxins, there was the potential for overall balance. But now, in the twentieth century, and particularly in the last fifty years, we are exposed to radiation, various chemicals, pesticides, and other stresses that cause electrons to become dislodged from their orbit in the atom. This onslaught results in too many free radicals for the system to handle.

There are a multitude of medical and scientific papers on free-radical-fighting antioxidants and books discussing them in mind-boggling detail. The purpose here is to provide information helpful in maintaining health. So, to save you time and to provide key data clearly, the following section on free-radical-fighting supplements is simplified to the essential facts. For the documenting medical references see the resource sections of Part IV.

▲

"In a 100 nation study on the quality of health, the U.S. was #1 in 1900, #1 in 1943 and #100 in 1992."
—U.S. Public Health Statistics

▲

There are two ways to fight free radical damage:

1. Reduce the causes of the overproduction of free radicals.
2. Supply additional sources of free radical scavengers.

ANTIOXIDANTS

As we have seen, there are two main kinds of free radical fighters: antioxidants, which are found in foods, and antioxidant enzymes, which are made by your body. Both may be taken as supplements. The antioxidant vitamins are vitamin A, or beta-carotene (which is transformed to vitamin A in the body), vitamin C, and vitamin E. They have chemistries that allow them to sacrifice an electron to neutralize the free radical and quench further free radical production. By this process their structure is changed.

Most antioxidants are supported by "co-worker" nutrient—co-factors—that can stabilize them after they've stabilized a free radical. This is known as the synergistic effect. For example, when vitamin E has donated an electron to neutralize a free radical, vitamin C can support it by donating an electron to the vitamin E. In this way, the antioxidants work together. Research has shown that the combination of vitamins A, C, and E and selenium was *more* effective than larger amounts of a single antioxidant. The whole *is* greater than the sum of the parts, so for optimum protection it is a good idea to combine all the antioxidants and their co-factors.

The recommended amount of an antioxidant would depend on the health of the individual, what their food intake is, and what amount of excess free radicals they are exposed to.

ANTIOXIDANT ENZYMES

Aside from the antioxidants just mentioned that are available from food as well as in supplements, there are antioxidant enzymes that are made by the body.

Enzymes are substances manufactured in your body that facilitate reactions. Digestive enzymes digest food. Metabolic enzymes facilitate various body processes. Among the metabolic enzymes are the antioxidant enzymes, which neutralize destructive free radicals.

The four antioxidant enzymes are superoxide dismutase (SOD), catalase, glutathione peroxidase, and methionine reductase.

When these antioxidant enzymes quench free radicals they do so without altering themselves. They do not lose or gain an electron in the act of counteracting free radicals. They just instigate changes. For example, catalase may take an unstable molecule and remove an oxygen atom and attach it to another oxygen molecule, producing a stable oxygen molecule. Catalase does not change and is ready to continue this job thousands of times.

The number of antioxidant enzymes is determined by the DNA in the cell and varies according to the number of free radicals. The capacity for producing these enzymes is contingent upon your nutritional status and your inherited potential— your genetics. Age may also be a factor; but this may be overcome by increasing nutrients to compensate for the possible deterioration usually associated with aging.

Aside from depending on your overall nutrient status, antioxidant enzymes require zinc, copper, selenium, manganese, and iron to work best. Sprouts and raw vegetables can reinforce the enzyme supply. Antioxidant precursors are available in supplement form and can be extremely useful in maintaining this critical balance and not allowing free radicals to become overwhelming. Glutathione peroxidase requires selenium and sulfur amino acids, which are found in cabbage family vegetables. SOD utilizes manganese, copper, and zinc. Catalase requires iron.

▲

"Vitamins promise to continue to unfold as one of the greatest and most hopeful stories of our day."
—"The Real Power of Vitamins," *Time*, April 6, 1992

▲

The antioxidant enzymes remove free radicals up to ten times faster than vitamins. This is important due to the fact that free radicals can do damage to a molecule in microseconds, resulting in a torrent of other free radical reactions.

We owe these efficient and quick antioxidant enzymes a debt of gratitude because without them we would suffer an increased rate of aging, and a variety of diseases. An inherited lack of antioxident enzymes causes accelerated aging and this is known as the disease progeria. At ten to fifteen years of age a person with progeria manifests all the symptoms of aging, including wrinkled skin, baldness, frailty, and heightened susceptibility to illness.

Of course, aside from utilizing all the antioxidants together, it is important to have all the necessary nutrients so that they become mutually supportive. This can be done by eating as well as possible from a selection of organically grown whole foods, and taking supplements that provide a broad-spectrum antioxidant defense. This will fill your needs thoroughly without creating problems from oversupplementing any particular antioxidant.

▲

"Let us report on what adding antioxidants and vitamin co-factors to our basic diet has meant to us personally. Our physical health has improved so dramatically over the past two or three years that our friends can hardly believe we are the same people."
—PHYLLIS AND EBERHARD KRONHAUSER, *Formula for Life*, 1989

▲

ANTIOXIDANT NUTRIENTS

Beta-carotene

Functions
Precursor to vitamin A, and is not toxic in large amounts
Protects the thymus gland
Helps to maintain the adrenal glands
Enhances wound healing
Reduces the incidents of heart attack, cancer, infections
Encourages the number of T cells
Defends against toxins
Retards aging
Maintains skin and mucous membranes

Deficiency Symptoms
Dry skin and hair
Susceptibility to infections
Night blindness
Risk of developing cataracts

Synergists
Choline, vitamins C, D, and E, the B complex vitamins and
   zinc

Dietary Sources
All green and yellow vegetables (especially leafy greens),
   squash and carrots, apricots

Amount
   RDA for beta-carotene is 3 mg or 5,000 IU of vitamin A.
I recommend 5,000 to 10,000 IU or 6 mg of beta-carotene to
maximize the protective benefits of this antioxidant. To counter
viruses in states of immune depletion, high amounts of beta-
carotene have been tested with good results.

▲

"People with low levels of vitamin A and E
are nearly twice as likely to need cataract
surgery as those with high levels."
—*New York Times*, December 6, 1992

▲

Vitamin E

Functions
Aids heart and circulation
Protects against toxins
Helps to prevent blood clots
Boosts immunity
Prevents damage to cell walls
May help prevent cataracts

Deficiency Symptoms
Skin disorders
Clogging of arteries
Cramps in calf of leg
Decreased production of antibodies

Synergists
Inositol, manganese, selenium, vitamins A, C, and B
    complex

Dietary Sources
Vegetable oils, cabbage, spinach, asparagus, leafy green
    vegetables

Amount
RDA: 30 IU
Protective: 50–800 IU daily

▲

"As an antioxidant, Vitamin C is effective,
together with Vitamin E in protecting cell
membranes against damage by oxidation."
—LINUS PAULING, Ph.D.

▲

Vitamin C

Functions
Supports the immune system and enhances resistance
Strengthens the blood vessels
Detoxifies
Essential for collagen production
Protects against heart disease
Helps build red blood cells

Blocks uptake of some radioactive elements
Maintains the adrenal gland

Deficiency Symptoms
Bleeding gums
Tendency to bruise easily
Scurvy
Susceptibility to infection

Synergists
The bioflavinoids, especially hesperidin and pycongenol,
    and all other vitamins

Dietary Sources
Especially high in leafy green vegetables and citrus fruits

Amount
RDA: 60 mg
Protective: 1,000–10,000 mg daily
In case of infection, accidental poisoning, insect bite or
    illness, increase to 1,000 every hour or half hour
    depending on circumstances and then decrease slowly
    to maintenance level.

Some doctors are using large amounts of vitamin C intrave-
nously to counteract depleted conditions with good results.

ANTIOXIDANT CO-FACTORS

Glutathione

Glutathione is an amino acid (protein) that is made in the
body and is supplied by foods.

Functions
A detoxifying agent
Helps repair the liver
Supports both the antioxidants and the antioxidant enzymes
Can "recycle" vitamins A and C, so it has a sparing effect
    on these vitamins

Deficiency Symptoms
Weak immunity

Synergists
The amino acids glycine, cysteine, and glutamic acid

Dietary Sources
In protein foods

Amounts
Protective: 100 mg to 300 mg
There is no toxic level, so amounts up to 1,000 mg have
    been used

▲

> "The number of fatalities from major
> pharmaceutical drugs for the seven year period
> from 1983 to 1989 equals 2069. The total
> number of fatalities from vitamin supplements
> over the period of 1983 to 1989 is zero."
> —American Association of Poison Control
> Centers, as reported in *The Townsend*
> *Newsletter for Doctors*

▲

B Complex Vitamins

The B vitamins play a vital supporting role to the antioxidants.

Functions
They are necessary for:
   carbohydrate metabolism
   growth
   healthy skin, hair, and nails
   the nervous system, to counter stress

Deficiency Symptoms
Nervousness
Cracks in the corner of mouth
Skin problems
Water retention (usually caused by insufficient B_6)
Low energy
Insomnia

Synergists
The whole B complex together, vitamins C and E

Dietary Sources
All whole grains, vegetables, and beans

Amounts
RDA: B_1:1.4 mg; B_2:1.6 mg; B_3: 1.8 mg; B_6: 2.2 mg; B_{12}:
   3 mcg; folic acid:400 mcg
Protective: ranging from 5 mg to 50 mg; folic acid should
   be 400 mcg and pantothenic acid, the "stress" B
   vitamin for the adrenal glands, may vary up to 200 mg
   (best taken with vitamin C)

"When subjects suffer from selenium and
vitamin E double deficiencies, the oxidative

damage observed is more severe than with deficiency of either antioxidant alone.''
—DR. J. LI and DR. F. STRATMAN, *Journal of the American College of Nutrition* (11:79), February 1992

▲

Selenium

Function
Enhances utilization of vitamin E
Preserves tissue elasticity
Essential for the internally made free-radical-fighting
    enzyme glutathione peroxidase
Detoxifies pollution

Deficiency Symptoms
Premature aging
Arthritis
Dandruff
Impaired ability of antibodies to respond to infection

Synergists
Vitamins A and E

Dietary Sources
Amounts in foods vary according to the content in the soil;
    many areas are deficient
Nuts and seeds, whole grains, barley, brown rice, oats,
    broccoli, garlic, fish

Amount
RDA: no RDA established
Protective: 50–200 mcg

Zinc

Functions
They are necessary for:
protein synthesis
collagen formation
the thymus gland (along with B_6), where the T cells are
made
wound healing
mobilizing stored vitamin A from the liver
the enzyme SOD

Deficiency Symptoms
Loss of taste
Slow wound healing
White, cloudy spots on the fingernails (a telltale sign of zinc
deficiency)
Mental imbalance

Synergists
Vitamins A, B_6, C, and E

Dietary Sources
Whole grains, green vegetables, sea vegetables

Amount
RDA: 15 mg
Protective: 15 to 50 mg

▲

"In 1990 Americans spent $13.7 billion on
alternative health treatments, versus $12.8
billion on traditional medical care. The
alternative treatments include herbal medicine,
relaxation techniques, homeopathy,
chiropractic and acupuncture."
—*The New England Journal of Medicine,*
March 1993

▲

"In a study by gerontologist Dr. Richard Cutler, the life spans of many mammalian species, including man, were found to be directly proportional to the amount of SOD they contain."
—DURK PEARSON and SANDY SHAW, *Life Extension*, 1988

▲

ANTIOXIDANT ENZYMES

Superoxide Dismutase (SOD)

Functions
Removes superoxide free radicals
Protects body organs from the assault of free radicals
Counters damage of radiation and radiation sickness
Slows the aging process
Counters breakdown of synovial fluid and thus prevents arthritis
Reduces chance of getting degenerative diseases

Synergists
Manganese, zinc, and copper

Dietary Sources
Sprouted grains and seeds, green plants such as spinach, parsley, wheat grass—all must be eaten raw

Amount
RDA: none established
Protective: Add sprouts and raw vegetables to your diet

2 to 7 tablets of 1.5 million units of Cell Guard, which is a
   compressed whole food of all four antioxidant
   enzymes.

▲

"The enhanced production of free radicals and
insufficient protection by antioxidant enzymes
apparently promote the transition from chronic
HIV infection to active disease development."
—VALERY POLYAKOV, SIU *Biopreparat*,
Rostov on Don, Russia, 1992

▲

Catalase

Functions
Works with superoxide dismutase (SOD)
Prevents formation of other free radicals
Counters inflammations such as arthritis, bursitis, gout
Has benefits similar to superoxide dismutase

Synergists
Iron

Dietary Sources
Sprouts and raw vegetables
Catalase is depleted by too much milk, bleached flour
   products, or polished white rice

Amount
RDA: none established
Protective: Add sprouts and raw vegetables to your diet
2 to 7 tablets of 1.5 million units of Cell Guard, which is a
   compressed whole food of all four antioxidant
   enzymes.

Glutathione Peroxidase

Functions
Quenches various types of free radicals
Protects the liver
Protects collagen and the skin
Helps remove brown pigment spots (age spots)

Synergists
Glutathione, selenium, cysteine, all the sulfur-containing
    amino acids such as in the cabbage family vegetables,
    vitamins C and E

Sources
Proteins, selenium-rich foods such as whole grains, garlic,
    broccoli

Amount
RDA: none established
Protective: Add sprouts and raw vegetables to your diet
2 to 7 tablets of 1.5 million units of Cell Guard, which is a
    compressed whole food of all four antioxidant
    enzymes.

Methionine Reductase

Functions
Quenches the most reactive free radical, the hydroxyl
    radical
Counters chemical poisoning
Counters effects of radiation exposure
Counters stress

Synergists
Spectrum of proteins and minerals

Dietary Sources
Live seed sprouts such as sunflowers, lentils, mung beans,
and raw green vegetables (see Part III for sprouting
directions)

Amounts
RDA: none established
Protective: Add sprouts and raw vegetables to your diet
2 to 7 tablets of 1.5 million units of Cell Guard, which is a
compressed whole food of all four antioxidant
enzymes.

ANTIOXIDANT ENZYMES

Free radical damage can be prevented if sufficient antioxidant enzymes are present to overcome the free radicals. For
insurance, consistent with caution in view of today's environment, consider taking an antioxidant enzyme supplement. The
Biotec Foods company in Hawaii makes one that contains one
quart of sprouts in each tablet and provides the nutritional
precursors to maintain good antioxidant enzyme levels. The
sprouts used are germinated from organically grown wheat.
The water is removed without harming the nutritional factors
in the sprouts, which are coated to retain availability in the
most receptive part of the digestive tract. This product, called
Cell Guard, has been shown to enhance the body's ability to
produce the antioxidant enzymes in the amounts required.

Research presented at the annual meeting of the American
Association for the Advancement of Science in Chicago in
February 1992 showed that adjustments to the gene that regulates the production of SOD (superoxide dismutase) could
vastly alter the life span of fruit flies, doubling their longevity.

Of relevance to our times, the Biotec company did a research project in Russia focusing on whether Cell Guard antioxidant enzymes would improve the health status of people contaminated with radioactive fallout from the accident at the Chernobyl nuclear plant. Their report concluded: "Subjects taking Cell Guard showed diminished cesium contamination, improved immune function, increased antioxidant activity, and increased attention span."

In a study conducted by Dr. Peter Rothschild including ten people between 67 and 76 years of age who took six tablets of Cell Guard for two weeks and three tablets for two weeks, the blood tests found a 230 percent increase in the levels of the antioxidant enzyme superoxide dismutase over pretest levels. Other clinical trials found improvement in symptoms such as inflammation and soreness of joints, and fatigue.

A CARROT A DAY KEEPS THE WRINKLES AWAY

Of course, a carrot alone won't do too much, but carrots along with the other antioxidants will retard wrinkling. All the above listed antioxidants and antioxidant enzymes work together to keep your skin from wrinkling. Free radicals cause what they call "cross-linking," which means that molecules are connected that should not be, and gradually cause what we see as wrinkles. As cosmetic chemistry expert Rebecca James puts it: "When free radicals attach to the connective tissues they hook the tiny fibers of collagen and elastin together. This process, known as cross-linking, prevents the fibers from moving freely, and wrinkling results." Fighting free radicals will slow this process, as well as slowing overall signs of aging. It also helps eliminate toxins, which results in a sense of well-being, which translates to a more energetic and youthful spirit and appearance. What more could we ask for?

There are many foods besides carrots with healing and health-building properties. Among them are two, garlic and blue-green algae, that are especially dependable, available, and easy to take as supplements to your food intake, a supportive insurance plan to guarantee that you win the fight against free radicals.

GARLIC

Garlic has been used since ancient times as a folk remedy for a variety of ailments. Dating back to 3000 B.C., garlic was used as a medicine by the Egyptians, Greeks, Indians, Romans, Babylonians, and Chinese. An Egyptian papyrus dated about 1500 B.C. lists twenty-two therapeutic formulas containing garlic as a remedy for ailments, including infections and tumors.

Garlic, a member of the lily family, contains dozens of sulfur compounds, which feed your antioxidant enzyme system, and it is through this mechanism that it fights free radicals.

Studies have demonstrated a multitude of protective health benefits of garlic. Clinical studies in China showed that feeding garlic to patients led to increased activity of immune cells. A nutritional study found that Kyolic (a form of commercially prepared garlic) helped eliminate the yeast *Candida albicans*. American epidemiological studies have shown that garlic may modulate tumor activity. It is reported to have the ability to counteract toxins in the form of heavy metals and radiation. By virtue of its antioxidant powers it has been found to be effective in inhibiting the damage of many major diseases. According to studies, it has antibacterial, antifungal, antiviral, and antiatherosclerotic properties. In *Garlic* (1986), Robert

Lin, Ph.D., sums up garlic's benefits: "Uniquely beneficial to modern man, garlic lowers the blood lipid levels, reduces the tendency of blood clotting, and may decrease cardiovascular risk. It also provides protection against free radicals and pollution."

KYOLIC

Too much raw garlic can have side effects such as stomach disorders and anemia. However, garlic that is aged has no such side effects. The safest and most effective garlic supplement and the only one proven to be an antioxidant goes by the trade name Kyolic. Kyolic is put through a twenty-month cold-aging process that accentuates the garlic's sulfur compounds and health-building properties, and by which it becomes deodorized. So there is no fear of garlic breath that will keep away vampires—and others. This is the only aged garlic extract that is organically grown.

▲

"This study demonstrated that Kyolic garlic extract enhanced elimination of candida albicans in animals systematically infected with this organism."
—P. TADI and R. TEEL, PH.D., "Anticandidal Potentials of Garlic," *International Clinic Nutrition Review*, 1990

▲

Studies Using Kyolic
Many studies have been done using Kyolic aged garlic extract, showing many beneficial results, among them:

- Antioxidant properties
- Detoxifying properties, including ridding the body of heavy metals
- Protection from radiation and pollution
- Lowering of cholesterol
- Protecting the liver
- Stimulating the production of T cells
- Antistress and antifatigue properties
- Counters bacteria, viruses, and fungi
- Effective against candida overgrowth
- Enhanced natural killer cells in people with AIDS
- Promotes growth of friendly bacteria in intestinal tract
- Enhances utilization of vitamin C
- Enhances vitamin E properties

Amount

Take Kyolic supplements, four to six 300 mg capsules daily, as a basic amount; in special cases such as illness or increased exposure to toxins, increase to eight to twelve capsules daily.

BLUE-GREEN ALGAE

Algae is one of the first life-forms on the planet. It has been used as an important food source by the Mayan and Aztec civilizations and by the people of China, Japan, Indonesia, Peru, and Ecuador. Algae is a primitive life form, but it is brilliantly efficient at photosynthesizing light and carbon dioxide from the air to make a high-energy package of proteins, carbohydrates, fats, nucleic acids (DNA and RNA), vitamins, and chlorophyll. Algae provides almost all the raw materials you need in a compact, clean, and easily assimilable form. Its nutrients are very densely packed, so even small amounts in your diet are beneficial. Its cleansing properties help to reduce free radicals. Its nutrients help to build free-radical-fighting antioxidants and antioxidant enzymes.

Algae contains a host of beneficial components: beta-carotene; minerals, including iron and magnesium; B vitamins, including B_{12}; proteins that are especially assimilable; neuro-peptides, which fortify the neurotransmitters in the brain so that the communication from brain to body and vice versa is optimum; chlorophyll, which detoxifies and fights free radicals; and raw materials for the synthesis of necessary molecules, including vitamin E.

Because it is a complete food, your body uses the health-building resources in algae more effectively than in vitamin supplements.

▲

"The most light filled foods are the blue green algae and organically grown fruits and vegetables."
—JACOB LIBERMAN, *Light, Medicine of the Future*, 1991

▲

KINDS OF ALGAE

Spirulina and chlorella are cultivated algaes. They are grown in huge pools with added nutrients. A particular species of algae referred to as blue-green algae (officially named apha-nizemon flos-aquae) grows naturally in a high-mineral mountainous lake in Oregon surrounded by 4,000 square miles of forest. It grows wild. It is enhanced by the unusually rich mineral water and the high-altitude clear sunshine. Once it is harvested it is freeze-dried to maintain its potency.

A variety of studies have shown that blue-green algae aids in better digestion, wound healing, improved vision, detoxification of heavy metals like lead and mercury, inhibiting growth of bacteria and yeast, normalizing the T cell count, countering the harmful effects of radiation, and supporting antioxidant enzymes. It is thought that the most beneficial aspects of algae might relate to as yet undiscovered ingredients in the algae.

Amount

Three to six capsules of blue-green algae are an average amount, more or less according to individual needs. (See Part IV Resources for more information on blue-green algae.)

ZINC AND VITAMIN B_6: TWO NUTRIENTS THAT ENHANCE THE THYMUS GLAND AND T CELLS

The two key nutrients that the thymus gland (an important part of the immune system) must have are the mineral zinc and the vitamin B_6. They work together to fortify the thymus so that it can do its function, which is to create T cells out of white blood cells. Circulating white blood cells go through the thymus and become T cells. If the necessary nutrients are missing, the T cell production will be limited and their maintenance job will be reduced accordingly.

Reasons for Reduced Availability of Zinc
Soil depletion
Food processing removes zinc
Stress increases the need for zinc
Excess alcohol
Excess copper reduces zinc

How to Ensure Availability
Eat whole grains, beans, and cabbage, and take a
    supplement
Supplement with 15–50 mg daily

Reasons for Reduced Availability of B$_6$
It is not in refined foods—it is processed out and not
    replaced
Stress depletes B$_6$
Birth control pills destroy B$_6$
High-fat, high-meal diets increase requirements
Antibiotics
Excess alcohol

How to Ensure Availability
Eat whole grains
Supplement with 10 to 100 mg daily

SOME MEDICATIONS DEPLETE NUTRIENTS

It is important to be aware that many medications (and
inert ingredients in some medications) can cause a depletion
of nutrients, often those needed for fighting free radicals.

Medication	Nutrients That Are Depleted
Alcohol	Magnesium, vitamin B complex, vitamins C, D, E, and K
Antacids	Calcium, phosphorus, vitamins A, B complex, and D
Anti-arrhythmic	Choline, pantothenic acid, potassium, vitamin K
Antibiotics	B vitamins, vitamin K

MEDICATION	NUTRIENTS THAT ARE DEPLETED
Anticonvulsant	Calcium, folic acid, riboflavin, vitamin K
Anti-inflammatory	Folic acid, vitamin C, iron
Antihistamines	Vitamin C
Antihypertensive	Potassium, magnesium, calcium, riboflavin, B_6, folic acid, phenylalanine
Aspirin	Calcium, folic acid, iron, potassium, B vitamins, vitamins A and C
Beta-blockers	Choline, chromium, pantothenic acid
Caffeine	Biotin, inositol, potassium, thiamine, zinc
Corticosteroid	Calcium, vitamins A, B_6, C, and D, potassium, zinc
Dilantin	Vitamin D
Diuretics	Calcium, iodine, magnesium, potassium, riboflavin, vitamin C, zinc
Estrogen	Folic acid, vitamin B_6
Gout medications (Allopurinol)	Iron
Laxatives (excluding herbs)	Potassium and other minerals, beta-carotene, vitamins A, D, and K
Coronary vasodilator	Niacin, selenium, pantothenic acid, vitamins C and E
Penicillin	Niacin, vitamin B_6
Phenobarbital	Folic acid, vitamins B_6, B_{12}, D, and K
Prednisone	Potassium, vitamins B_6 and C, zinc
Tranquilizers	Riboflavin

HERBS

Herbs have existed since before there were people. When animals and humans came along they used herbs to their benefit. Ancient cultures had a valuable healing resource in herbs and an extensive knowledge of herbal medicine developed. The intrinsic healing properties of herbs were recognized and utilized.

Traditional cultures passed on their herbal lore through generations until the twentieth century. Modern medicine organized the sale and distribution of single-focus drugs that suppress, rather than heal. The more generalized, tonic, and health-building herbs took a back seat.

Recently the efficacy of herbs has been established by clinical research and there is a resurgence of respect. As a result, many high-quality herbal preparations are now available. It is best to seek guidance from a knowledgeable practitioner or, even better, to develop your own herbal knowledge. See Part IV for a list of resources for herbal studies. Herbs can assist in countering free radicals by supplying nutrients, by detoxifying, and by strengthening the immune system. Some herbs also have antioxidant properties.

▲

"Herbs are nature's gift of medicines to humankind."
—LAURENCE E. BADGLEY, M.D.,
Energy Medicine, 1985

▲

Following is a list of some herbs that help in the fight against free radicals.

Burdock Root

A good herb to eliminate toxins, as it has strong cleansing properties. It is known as a blood purifier.

Yellow Dock Root

A marvelous cleanser for the lymphatic system and also a blood cleanser.

Red Clover

Known to kill certain bacteria and viral and fungal infections. It is a blood purifier containing many minerals.

Dandelion

A cleansing diuretic that stimulates the liver to eliminate toxins. It is mentioned in many ancient documents.

Ginkgo Biloba

An antioxidant and also an aid to circulation and to the nervous system. It is the leading phytomedicine prescribed worldwide and ranks in the top three "best-sellers" in France and Germany.

Echinecea

A great support for the immune system. It has antibiotic and antiviral properties. Research has shown it is a boon for T cells and white blood cells.

Silymarin (Milk Thistle)

A premier liver detoxifier and rejuvenator. Good liver function is crucial for a healthy immune system. Research shows *Silymarin* inhibits free radical damage.

Alfalfa

A powerful cleanser and remineralizer. It can be taken in tablet form. Some of the best are made by Dr. Bernard Jensen.

Astragalus

An excellent tonic for the immune system and a barrier for toxic chemicals.

Essiac

An herbal tea based on an old Canadian Indian recipe. The name Essiac is from the name of the Canadian nurse (Rene Caisse—Essiac spelled backward) who discovered it when she observed amazing improvement in one of her patients. This can be ordered from: Pure Hart Nutrition, (212) 966-5687.

Green Tea

Used for years in Japan and was recently discovered to be an excellent antioxidant.

Of course, the complete range of necessary nutrients is ideal to ensure a strong fight against free radicals. This can be attained by eating a broad variety of organic whole foods (see Chapter 3) and by supplementing the above antioxidants and occasionally other nutrients as necessary.

Following are a few special supplements to consider.

▲

"Deficiencies are what lead to the uptake of radioactive elements."
—SARA SHANNON, *Diet for the Atomic Age*, 1987

▲

SOME SUPPORTIVE SUPPLEMENTS

Co-Enzyme Q10

This is essential to the production of energy in the metabolism of foods. It is likened to a cellular sparkplug. It can be synthesized in the body, but it is often in low supply. It is effective as a free radical fighter.

Pycnogenol

A bioflavinoid (part of the vitamin C family) extracted from the bark of the pine tree. It is a powerful free radical scavenger.

Kelp

A source of iodine, which is necessary for the thyroid gland to function well. Besides this, when sufficient natural iodine is eaten the body's tendency to absorb radioactive iodine-131 as an iodine source is reduced. This is an important and easy way of stopping the intake of one of the radioactive elements that are released from nuclear power plants. Radiation causes free radicals, so stopping this process before it happens is a good idea.

Other radioactive elements are kept out on the same principle. For example, if you have enough calcium in your body to fill its requirements, you will not absorb its related radioactive element, strontium-90. This is critical to understand, because if you know that you can reduce your absorption of modern ever-present man-made radiation, then you will be the more inspired to eat well. This principle does not afford infinite protection, so efforts also need to be made to reduce the source of the problem.

STABLE ELEMENTS THAT BLOCK THE UPTAKE OF THEIR RADIOACTIVE COUNTERPARTS

STABLE ELEMENT	RADIOACTIVE COUNTERPART
Calcium	Strontium-90
Iodine	Iodine-131
Iron	Plutonium-238, -239
Potassium	Cesium-137
Sulfur	Sulfur-35
Vitamin B_{12}	Cobalt-60
Zinc	Zinc-65

Essential Fatty Acids

Oils that cannot be synthesized by the body are referred to as essential fatty acids. Estimates say that about 80 percent of the population has a deficiency of essential fatty acids which are important because they are immune stimulants and provide necessary ingredients for immune activities. Fatty acids help to control viral infections, may improve skin problems, enhance immunity, have been shown to reduce cholesterol, and improve overall energy.

Good sources are fish, green vegetables, and oils such as flaxseed oil and walnut oil.

IMPROVE DIGESTION AND INTESTINAL HEALTH

Enzymes are a key to health. "You are what you eat" should be rephrased to "you are what you digest." The proteins, carbohydrates, fats, minerals, and vitamins in your food cannot be utilized as they are. They need to be activated by digestive enzymes, which act as catalysts to transform foods into useful energy. All raw foods in their natural state contain enzymes. But enzymes are killed by cooking at a heat above 120°F. Your body manufactures enzymes and there is a potential hitch here, too, if you are lacking in the necessary raw materials or there is a malfunction of the pancreas or liver. In addition, you may lack digestive enzymes because food is grown in enzyme deficient soil, your diet consists mostly of cooked or processed food, or because stress depletes your enzymes. To replenish your body's supply of enzymes, eat a generous amount of raw, organic fresh foods, and take digestive enzyme supplements to encourage assimilation of your foods.

INTESTINAL HEALTH

Your body's ability to absorb nutrients and at the same time reject toxins depends largely on the condition of the lining of the intestinal tract. This is kept optimum by emphasizing fresh vegetables and grains and high-fiber foods and avoiding processed foods, including white flour.

There are various intestinal cleansing programs that feature a fiber, usually a mixture of psyllium, pectin, and agar, to be taken along with herbs in a tablet.

Having selected free radical fighting foods and supplements, the next thing to do is to incorporate an exercise program, and the following chapter gives some suggestions.

CHAPTER 5

Exercise—Pumping Immunity

"It isn't like I've got some amazing secret that nobody else has. When I don't exercise, I look like hell."   —*Cher*

*W*ith the explosion of interest in fitness that emerged out of the New Frontier of the Kennedy administration in the 1960s, followed by the Jane Fonda aerobics enthusiasm in the 1970s and 1980s, and the blooming interest in walking as a health restorer, it would seem that Americans are a physically active bunch. But this is not true. At a meeting of fitness experts and the Centers for Disease Control in the spring of 1993, it was announced that the impression that more Americans are engaged in physical activity is wrong. In fact, they reported, almost 60 percent of Americans over age eighteen were physically inactive. The Director of the CDC, Dr. Walter Dowdle, said: "Only 22 percent of Americans are active today to levels recommended for good health benefits" (quoted in *The New York Times*, July 30, 1993).

MODERATION

Research has shown that moderate exercise can enhance the immune system and overall health, while too much exercise may generate excess free radicals. Exercise increases the body's need for oxygen and so more free radicals are formed. Studies at the Cleveland Clinic by immunologist Dr. Leonard Calabrese showed that moderate exercise, such as forty-five minutes of walking or bicycling at about 60 percent of maximum heart rate, four or five times a week, may lead to fewer colds and flus. Studies on overtraining conducted by exercise scientist Dr. David Nieman found that runners who ran sixty miles a week or more got twice as many respiratory infections as those who ran twenty miles a week. It is also known that marathoners are prone to develop infections the week after a race.

Normally, the amount of oxygen consumed in moderate exercise is not a problem. But intense workouts and the overtraining of endurance athletes require high levels of oxygen, which result in increased amounts of harmful free radicals. Heavy training may also cause the breakdown of body fats and the release of free-radical-causing toxins stored in the fat. If unchecked, these free radicals can cause damage to muscle tissue, be harmful to overall health, and result in early aging.

ANTIOXIDANT PROTECTION

Various researchers have found that antioxidants have the power to protect from exercise-generated free radicals. Mohsen Meydani, in studies at the Research Center for Aging at Tufts University, found evidence that vitamin E supplements can counteract the excess free radicals brought about from heavy exercise. According to a study done at the Sports Science and

Fitness Research Center in Melbourne, Australia, endurance athletes who took 1000 IU of vitamin E and 1000 milligrams of vitamin C daily had 25 percent less tissue damage.

The key point to make here is that a certain amount of exercise is necessary and beneficial. Yet, *too much* can be detrimental. Unless you have an abundance of free radical fighters, a very heavy exercise program will leave you in a state of weakened immunity. You can compensate by utilizing extra supplements *or* you can do moderate exercise with extra supplements and be assured of the benefits of exercise without its extra stresses.

▲

"To keep the body in good health is a
duty. . . . Otherwise we shall not keep our
mind strong and clear."
—BUDDHA

▲

Benefits of Exercise

Increases respiration and oxygen utilization

Increases oxygen level, which creates an unreceptive environment for virus, and improves digestion and assimilation

Increases perspiration, which releases toxins

Increases circulation, which carries nutrients to eliminate toxins

Pumps the lymph system, which facilitates the immune function

Stimulates endorphin production

Cleanses the arteries by mobilizing fats (exercise combined with a low-fat diet is the essence of the Pritikin Plan for cardiovascular health)

Increases muscle to fat ratio

Improves heart efficiency, resulting in cardiovascular fitness

Lowers blood pressure (58 million Americans have high
blood pressure)

Improves levels of cholesterol

Strengthens bones (osteoporosis affects 24 million
Americans)

Reduces anxiety and stress

Imparts a tranquilizing effect

Increases energy

Improves your self-concept

Promotes healing and ability to detoxify

Increases production of lymphocytes, which fight bacteria

Produces antibodies for protection

Slows growth of cancer

Makes it impossible for virus to live in an oxygen
environment

Combined with low-fat diet can cause regression of
arteriosclerosis

Recent evidence suggests that exercise stimulates the secretion of morphinelike chemicals in the brain called endorphins. They have a painkilling effect, increase sense of well-being (causing what is known as ''runner's high''), and also directly support the strong immune system that is needed to counteract free radicals. Researchers at Massachusetts General Hospital found that there is an over 100 percent increase in endorphins after just one hour of exercise. When we connect this knowledge with the recently discovered fact that there is a receptor site on the T cell—which is a *key* cell in the immune system—specifically made to connect with endorphins and to utilize their health-enhancing characteristics, it becomes clear that exercise is indispensable. Endorphins improve the power of T cells, and if only one hour of exercise creates more than

100 percent more endorphins, then there is all the more reason to figure out what exercise you prefer—and then do it!

While the blood system has a pump—the heart—the lymph system, however, does not. Exercise, movement, and stretching are what pump the lymph system. Deep breathing cleanses it.

Several studies have shown that both men and women over sixty who train with resistance machines several times a week can quickly double their strength. Researcher David Nieman, Ph.D., at Appalachian State University, studied the immune function of groups of women over seventy, those who exercise and those who don't. Of course those who exercise came out ahead. But the interesting finding was that the women over seventy who exercised one and a half hours a day were far ahead of thirty-year-old women who were sedentary. The elderly athletes had a higher level of natural killer cells, a type of immune cell. "The usual age-related decline in immune function was very nearly reversed in these lean and highly active women," says Nieman.

A study in the *Journal of the American Medical Association* in 1989 that observed 13,000 women of general good health in their forties found that the physically fit were three times less likely to die over the eleven-year period of the study.

One of the key benefits of exercise—such as breathing exercises, brisk walking, yoga, recreational exercise, or your preferred sport—is that it oxygenates the blood. You can also oxygenate the blood by increasing your intake of green foods, raw foods, and juices, and avoiding pollutants and electromagnetic radiation (which causes clumping of the red blood cells, thus slowing oxygen transport).

To get all the benefits of exercise, without the risks of *too much* exercise, exercise for thirty to ninety minutes five times a week, always warm up, and if you are doing heavy exercise, have a day of rest between workouts. Finish each exercise session with ten minutes of total relaxation lying on the floor, and, of course, maintain a low-fat diet, emphasizing grains and vegetables. Make sure you see a medical professional before undertaking any new exercise regime, and only increase duration and intensity gradually. Listen to your body—don't exercise if you have an infection or when you're feeling tired.

The three kinds of exercise everybody needs are aerobic, resistance strengthening, and flexibility. Flexibility exercises include yoga and stretching. Aerobic exercise, like brisk walking, increases your pulse. Resistance exercise builds bone density through the use of weights or body resistance (as in yoga and some martial arts).

Types of Exercise

AEROBIC	EVERYDAY ACTIVITY	RESISTANCE STRENGTH	FLEXIBILITY
walking	gardening	weight lifting	yoga
swimming	cleaning house	gymnastics	stretching
running	cutting lawn	calisthenics	tai chi
bike riding	shoveling snow	martial arts	
dancing		tai chi	
rope jumping			
stair climbing			
martial arts			
skiing			
boxing			
horseback riding			
golf			
soccer			
tennis			

AEROBIC

aerobics sessions
trampoline
rowing machine

There are four components of fitness. Cardiovascular fitness is the heart's ability to pump blood and transport and use oxygen. Muscular fitness is your body's muscular strength. Flexibility increases your ability to move joints freely. Body composition optimizes the ratio of body fat to muscle.

▲

"A sedentary life is the real sin against the Holy Spirit. Only those thoughts that come by walking have any value."
—NIETZSCHE

▲

WALKING

Have you overdone running? Are you fed up with jogging? Are you a person who does little exercise? Everyone can benefit from brisk walking. Give walking a try! Statistics show that 69 million Americans walked for exercise in 1991, making it one of the fastest growing activities. Walking builds immunity without the negative of the musculoskeletal stress of running. It gives you aerobic activity, strengthening activity, improves circulation, and at the same time offers the great pluses of full-spectrum light (explained in Chapter 7) and outdoor oxygen and the aesthetics of nature if you walk outdoors.

Studies on the Benefits of Walking

A study at the Institute for Aerobics Research in Texas (*Journal of the American Medical Association*, November 3, 1989), found that those people who were in a moderate state of fitness fared almost as well as those in a high state of fitness in terms of mortality during the eleven years of the study. The author of the study, Dr. Steven Blair, suggests the following:

For Moderate Fitness
WOMEN:
1. Walk 2 miles in under 30 minutes at least 3 days a week. Or:
2. Walk 2 miles in 30–40 minutes 5–6 days a week.

MEN:
1. Walk 2 miles in under 27 minutes at least 3 days a week. Or:
2. Walk 2 miles in 30–40 minutes 6–7 days a week.

For High Fitness
WOMEN:
1. Walk 2 miles in under 30 minutes 5–6 days a week.

MEN:
1. Walk 2½ miles in under 37½ minutes 6–7 days a week.

Another study at the Institute of Aerobics Research (*Journal of the American Medical Association*, December 1992) confirms that a certain amount of moderate exercise is beneficial. Dr. John Duncan, who authored this study, says: "Train, don't strain," and points out the beneficial effects of moderate fitness are assured with a frequency of four to five days per week and a duration of about forty-five minutes. If you want to increase benefits go for the increase in duration rather than intensity.

It works the other way, as well: a study at Harvard and Stanford found that men who did not exercise regularly have an 85 percent higher risk of death due to cardiovascular disease, an overall death rate from any cause 63 percent higher, and die four to five years earlier than those who are active.

▲

"We are underexercised as a nation. We look instead of play. We ride instead of walk. Our existence deprives us of the minimum of physical activity essential for healthy living."
—John F. Kennedy, 1960

▲

Get Started Walking Briskly

See how long it takes you to walk a mile—probably between fifteen and twenty minutes if you are a beginner. Build it up from there. You can measure by your car or a pedometer. In the some cities ten blocks is about a mile. The recommended heart rate is about 60 to 90 percent of your maximum heart rate. To find your maximum:

subtract your age (in years) from 220, and
multiply by .6 and .9 to get the range.

$$
\begin{array}{rr}
\text{For example:} & 220 \\
& -40 \\
\hline
& 180 \qquad 180 \\
& \times .6 \qquad \times .9 \\
\hline
& 108 \qquad 162 \\
\end{array}
$$

So target range is between 108 and 162.

Make up your mind to walk a certain number of times per week. Make a date with yourself. Write the appointment in your datebook. Keep it.

You will need a good pair of shoes. Running shoes are not appropriate for walking, nor are shoes with no support. Athletic shoe stores carry shoes specifically designed for walking. These are ideal. Make sure they have firm support and plenty of room for the toes.

▲

"Unhappy businessmen, I am convinced,
would increase their happiness more by
walking six miles every day than by any
conceivable changes in philosophy."
—BERTRAND RUSSELL, 1960

▲

Brisk Walking Benefits

To get the most out of walking, swing the arms fully with your stride, stand tall with the body aligned, and place feet firmly facing forward, neither pointed in or out. Maintain a steady pace—don't stop and start—and walk continuously for at least forty-five minutes. Finally, choose the most beautiful area near where you live, and if you like, walk with a pal.

Levels of Walking

strolling
brisk walking—about 3 miles in 45 minutes
aerobic walking—10- to 14-minute mile
race walking—10-minute mile or less

Ideas for Walking

Enjoy a nature walk in a state park.
Walk on a beach.
Find the most appealing lane or road near you.
Choose an area a short drive away and make an outing
    every Saturday or Sunday.
As a last resort go early to a nearby mall and walk briskly
    before customers arrive.

Walking Is for Everyone!

It adds variety, aesthetics of scenery, has no stress on
joints, and provides a cardiovascular workout, oxygen, and
light. It is vigorous yet nonstressful.

▲

"Enjoying Yoga, I am indeed most happy."
—MILAREPA, Tibetan poet, 11th century

▲

YOGA

Yoga is an art, a philosophy, and a discipline. The aspects
of yoga most known in the West are the physical postures
that, when practiced over time, result in impressive physical,
mental, psychological, and spiritual development in its practitioners. With yoga, you can relax, revitalize, reshape, and
release.

Yoga benefits the immune system as well as the glandular
system, including the lymph system, the thyroid gland, and the

pituitary gland. It enhances flexibility, increases strength and tone and endurance, and gives a sense of youthfulness.

Even athletes who run or work out with weights also need to stretch. Muscles and ligaments may have shortened. Yoga stretches are ideal for them.

▲

"One technique to help you with exercise is called 'visualization.' It is the art of picturing in your mind the results you would like to see happen, and using these images to focus all your energies on attaining your goals."
—Arnold Schwarzenegger

▲

RECOMMENDED DAILY EXERCISE ROUTINE

This daily exercise routine is a combination of martial arts, yoga, and calisthenics. It will take about twenty-five minutes, plus the fifteen-minute complete relaxation at the end. If you do not have much time, do exercises one through nine, and then lie down for a five-minute relaxation. Try to do this routine in addition to your walking. If time is too pressing, alternate days.

Do not push yourself. Some of these stretches and poses may be difficult at first. Ease into them, do them gently, and you will begin to see improvement quickly. If any position is painful, don't do it. As always, you should check with your doctor before embarking on a new exercise program.

Suggestions:
1. First thing in the morning is best, before eating.
2. Prepare a place.

3. Have a mat, a rug, or yoga mat.
4. Be sure there are no disturbances.

This exercise routine will help you to require less sleep. After a certain point, the amount of sleep you need is determined by the level of toxins in your body. This exercise routine will increase oxygen and flexibility, and pump the cleansing lymph system to eliminate toxins. After a week or so you will observe the changes.

DRY BRUSH MASSAGE

In combination with these exercises, follow them with a dry brush massage before your shower:

Purchase a natural vegetable bristle bath brush
Before your shower, brush your dry skin with this brush, in
    a circular fashion, from toes toward head.
Brush lightly, yet firmly.
Do this for three to five minutes, then shower.

This massage removes top skin cells, rejuvenates skin, eliminates toxins, and assists the kidneys to do their job—some naturopaths refer to the skin as the "third kidney."

1. SHOULDER ROLL
    Stand relaxed, knees slightly bent
    Lift shoulders—up, and back, and down
    Inhale up—exhale down

Do: Repeat 6 times

 Lift shoulders—up, FRONT, and down

 Inhale up, exhale down

Do: Repeat 6 times

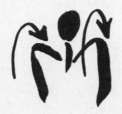

2. NECK ROLL

 Stand relaxed, knees slightly bent

 Drop chin to chest, exhale

 Drop left ear to left shoulder, inhale

 Drop head back, exhale

 Drop right ear to right shoulder, inhale

 Drop head forward, exhale

Do: Repeat 3 times to the left and 3 times to the right

 Do slowly and thoughtfully

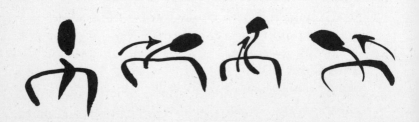

3. **SIDE BEND**
   Clasp hands overhead, palms facing the ceiling

   Stretch up, relax pelvis down

   Lean to left, exhale, hold 2–3 seconds

   Return to center, inhale

   Lean to right, exhale, hold 2–3 seconds

   Return to center, inhale

Do: Repeat 3 times

   Do slowly and thoughtfully, inhale yourself to center

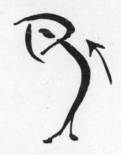

4. **MARTIAL ART SQUAT**
   Stand relaxed, feet 3 feet apart

   Raise arms overhead, palms facing forward, inhale

   Lower arms in front, palms facing down, exhale

   At the same time sink slowly down, pelvis tucked under until in squatting position, heels on floor, knees spread, arms straight ahead, palms facing down

   Hold for 5 seconds while finishing the exhale

   Start to inhale while pushing down on heels and raise up

Raise up straight and lift arms overhead

Lower arms to side while exhaling

Do: *Repeat 2–5 times*

Duration of squatting about 15–20 seconds, raising up about 15–20 seconds

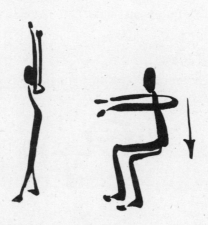

5. TWIST

Stand relaxed, feet about 18 inches apart

Feel as if you are suspended from the sky, with pelvis sinking down

Place hands in front of your chest

Twist to your right, letting your right hand stretch out around to the right with the palm facing up

Let your head turn to the right

Exhale as you turn and hold the twist for 2–3 seconds

Return to the center as you inhale

Repeat on the other side

Do: Repeat 5 times to each side

Important points:

Keep your mind focused on the twist

Keep your pelvis facing forward, only the top of the
body turning

Create maximum torsion at the point of twisting

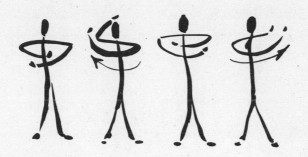

6. **ARM LIFTS**

Stand relaxed, knees slightly bent, neck suspended

Bend arms at elbows and let hang straight out at side,
even with shoulders

Lift upper arm several inches 10 times

Move elbows forward and do same

Move elbows behind shoulder line, and do same

Do: Repeat 2–5 times

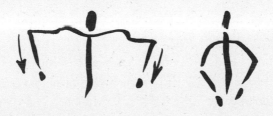

7. **ARM PRESS**
   Stand relaxed, knees slightly bent, neck suspended

   Place hands and forearms together, hands in front of
   face

   Open forearms outward with resistance, even to
   shoulder line

   Move arms as if against a force

   Repeat 10 times

Do: The same starting from arm open, even with shoulders

   Press arms together as if against a resistance

   Repeat 10 times

   Exhale with the tension

Do: 2 to 5 sets

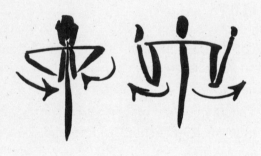

8. **DOWNWARD DOG**
   Place hands on floor about 3–4 feet in front of feet

   Fingers spread, arms with inside of elbow facing
   forward

Feet touching floor, tension in legs, head loose

Hold 20–30 seconds in upside-down V

Slowly move body forward, release out of V, bring chest forward into upward facing with chest facing forward, arms straight

Hold 20–30 seconds

Return to Downward Dog

Do: Repeat 2–5 times

9. **PLOUGH**

Lie on back

Slowly lift legs together vertical to floor—hold

Lift legs backward over head and touch toes to floor

Place hands for support on lower back

If can't reach floor, remain where comfortable

Hold 30 seconds

Do: Repeat 2–3 times

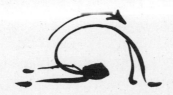

10. **FORWARD BEND**

Sit on floor, feet extended, legs together

Lift arms overhead, inhale

Slowly go forward over legs, exhale

Gently stretch where comfortable for you, hands may hold ankles

Release into the legs

Let go and sit up slowly

Hold 30 seconds to 2–3 minutes

Do: One time

Daily practice will improve the stretch, relax into the pose

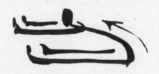

11. **SHOULDER STAND**

Lie on back

Lift legs overhead

Place hands on small of back and raise legs high over head

Hold legs straight, relaxed, with no tension, let blood flow down

Chin will touch chest

Relax breathing

Hold 30 seconds to 2–5 minutes

Release by lowering legs very slowly to the floor

Do: Repeat 1 time

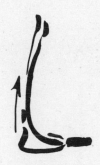

12. OPPOSITE LEG/ARM LIFT

Lie on floor on stomach with arms outstretched above
  your head

Lift right arm and left leg

Hold 5–10 seconds

Release to floor

Lift left arm and right leg

Hold 5–10 seconds

Release to floor

Do: Repeat 2 5 times

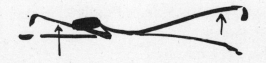

13. CRUNCH

Lie on back, put feet together on wall at a right angle to the wall

Place hands behind head

Using your abdominal muscles, lift your shoulders and upper back off the floor, exhale, hold

Relax down

Do: Repeat 20–50 times

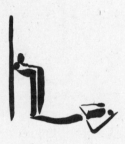

14. RELAXATION

Get a 6- to 8-inch inflatable rubber ball and place it between the shoulder blades, middle of the back

Relax lying over the ball, hands out to side (if you do not have a rubber ball, fold over some towels)

Lie with relaxation 1–2 minutes

Relax Pose

Lie on mat or carpet

Feet together, let them fall open

Hands 6 inches from body, palms up

Head relaxed

Eyes closed
Even breathing
Empty mind
Sink into floor
Float into clear blue sky
Remain 10–15 minutes

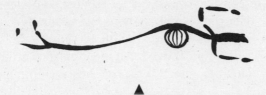

▲

"One who has this precious knowledge [of breathing] is unique, because he or she knows the technique of working with the body, mind and consciousness in the most efficient way." —HARISH JOHARI, *Breath, Mind and Consciousness*, 1989

▲

BREATHING

We seem to take breathing for granted. But breathing has a great influence on physical and mental functions, so it is worth some extra attention.

The breathing exercises in this section will help you increase awareness and perception, tune brain waves to the beneficial alpha waves, improve your mood by producing endorphins, calm your response to stress, reduce production of debilitating adrenaline, tone your lymph system, and generally keep your vital organs in a healthy state. The life force, or "chi" as they say in the East, can be utilized and inner balance achieved by slow, conscious breathing, which causes the life energy to travel through the body providing relaxation and rejuvenation.

Oxygen is a key to good health. Nobel Prize winner Dr. Otto Warburg found in 1925 that cancer cells flourish in an *absence* of oxygen. When there is insufficient oxygen, carbon monoxide (CO) is formed, which is *not* eliminated well, and is enervating to the body, resulting in less resistance to bacteria, toxins, and disease. Breathing exercises help keep a good supply of oxygen flowing throughout your body.

Breathing is a crucial link in the whole life cycle.

Breathing exercises help counteract the oxygen shortage your body may have, caused by shallow breathing, a sedentary lifestyle, a high-fat, high-protein diet, a nutrient deficient diet, cholesterol build up inside arteries, and diminishing sources of oxygen including trees and plankton.

▲

"While we practice conscious breathing, our thinking will slow down, and we can give ourselves a real rest."
—THICH NHAT HANH, *Peace Is Every Step*, 1991

▲

"[Yoga's breathing technique] purifies the nervous system and eliminates toxins from the body. This is not just Yoga wisdom; it's also scientific. Today, scientists know we normally take in only 500 cubic centimeters of air in a normal breath. By using deep breathing Yoga practices, we take in as much as 4000 cubic centimeters in one breath."
—SWAMI SATCHIDANANDA, *Contemplating Yoga*, 1991

▲

FOUR BREATHING PRACTICES

For all breathing exercises, breathe through the nose, be in the cleanest air possible, and don't do them just after eating.

STANDING BREATHING
This is an easy breathing exercise that's good to do several times during the day:

Stand up, arms relaxed at your sides

Raise hands in front of you and inhale slowly to a count of 6

Spread arms in a V overhead and inhale 2 more breaths while lifting muscles of upper chest

Drop arms down forcibly in front of you while exhaling and pull stomach back in toward spine

Do: Repeat 3 times

THE COMPLETE BREATH

Sit in a comfortable place

Relax, close eyes

Inhale through nose to a count of 4

Hold breath to a count of 8

Exhale through nose to a count of 12

Do: Repeat 10 times

▲

"Happiness is there if you know how to breathe and smile, because happiness can always be found in the present moment."
—THICH NHAT HANH, *Peace Is Every Step*, 1991

▲

BELLOWS BREATH

This is a dynamic way to cleanse the lungs, air out the system, recharge the body, and strengthen the abdomen:

Sit in a comfortable place with the spine straight

Inhale a small amount of air through the nose

Exhale by contracting the abdomen and forcing the air out through the nose

The attention is on the exhale, the inhale will be automatic

Keep a regular beat

Start with 10 exhalations, follow with a long inhale and slow exhale

Do: 3 sets of 10

Then increase to 3 sets of 30 breaths

Benefits: will cleanse blood, create higher voltage of nerve cells, increase circulation, detoxify

ALTERNATE NOSTRIL BREATHING
Sit in a comfortable place

Fold in the first 2 fingers of your right hand—leaving the thumb and last 2 fingers free (with these you close the left and the right nostril)

Count to 4

Inhale through the left nostril, hold with the two fingers

Hold, count to 8

Exhale right nostril, count to 4

Inhale right nostril, count to 4

Hold with the thumb, count to 8

Exhale left nostril, count to 4

Inhale left nostril, and hold and continue . . .

Benefits: will balance energy and, according to B.K.S. Iyengar, "increase radiance and beauty"

THREE HELPFUL HINTS

The following three procedures can really help your health, they are easy to do, and don't cost money!

Thump the Thymus

The thymus gland is located in the middle of your chest about an inch below your collarbone. The thymus makes

T cells, creating them out of white blood cells of the immune system; the T cells do important defense work in the body.

In *Maximum Life Span,* Dr. Roy Walford stresses the importance of the thymus: ''The thymus is the master gland of the immune system. It manufactures a family of hormones which regulate the growth of a sizable part of the immune system. The thymus gland may be a primary pacemaker for aging.'' The thymus depends on certain nutrients, but it can also be benefited by circulation and energy and this can be enhanced by thumping: take your fist and gently but firmly thump this area. You can thump the thymus several times during the day. It's certainly an inexpensive and quick therapy, so give it a try!

The Slant Board

The slant board is a board you lie on at an angle so that your head is lowered. The foot end of the board should be raised eighteen inches. This board can be made yourself or bought from an exercise equipment supplier.

Twenty minutes daily on the slant board will help blood circulation, counteract gravity, and energize the pituitary gland in the head as well as the thyroid in the neck. These are ''master glands'' and will influence the rest of the body systems. The slant board also energizes the liver, which does more than 400 jobs in the body. Dr. Bernard Jensen, a respected naturopath and healer, calls the slant board ''God's gift.''

You can make your own version of the slant board by putting phone books, the equivalent of six to eight inches, one on top of the other, placing a thick towel or blanket over them, and then lying with your behind on the phone books and head and shoulders releasing onto the floor. Lie like this for ten to twenty minutes to derive great benefit.

Reflexology

Reflexology is pressure-point massage for the feet. The foot is the pathway to the rest of the body. Similar to acupuncture, the principle is that there are connections from points on the foot to all the body organs, and by pressing a certain area you can affect the related organ. Organs that are "located" in these areas can be stimulated by pressing their various reflex points. According to this ancient therapy, reflexology releases energy blocks and opens energy currents, thus encouraging optimum well-being.

You can give your own feet a reflexology treatment, or ask a friend. Press the area on the bottom of the foot with the side of the thumb. Visualize the area you want to heal. Hold for a few seconds, release, and press again. You can also rub over the spot while pressing deeply. If the area feels tender, this means it is related to an organ that is below par, so you know to give it extra attention. You can rub the feet lightly with some good oil, such as olive oil. Rest afterward to absorb the benefits. A reflexology treatment could last anywhere from 5 minutes to a half hour, depending on the time you have. A few minutes a day would be beneficial, or once a week for a longer period of time. If you sense an illness coming on, work on your feet.

See the map of the feet on the next page that shows all the main points and lists the key points to press to energize specific parts of the immune system.

Foot Reflexology

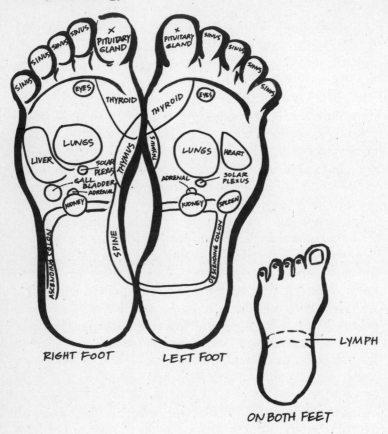

RIGHT FOOT   LEFT FOOT

ON BOTH FEET

To send energy to the immune system, press:

the spleen—on left foot

the liver—on right foot

the thymus—on both feet

the intestines (ascending and descending colons)—on both feet

lymphatic drainage—on both feet

brain and pineal—on both big toes

GOAL SETTING

The best way to get exercise (or any new habit) ingrained in your life is to make specific goals.

For example: Make a deal with yourself that you'll walk four miles or forty minutes, four or five times a week, and do ten minutes of stretching, and do five to ten minutes of breathing exercises daily. You can tailor the program to your needs and interests. Use a chart in your home or office, like the one that follows, to keep yourself on track.

LONG-RANGE HEALTH GOALS

FITNESS CHART

Health Goal for This Week

	Week 1	Week 2	Week 3	Week 4
Exercise				
Breathing				
Workout				
Gym				
Walking				
My sport				
Meditation				

CHAPTER 6
Mind over Stress

"The brain produces narcotics up to two hundred times stronger than anything you can buy on the street."
—*Deepak Chopra*

*I*n the modern world, we all face extremely high levels of stress, at least from time to time. Stress, when not controlled and counteracted, is a major factor in excess free radical production and health deterioration. The interaction of the mind and the body is crucial to good health, as this chapter details.

We now know everything is related. The earth we live on affects us—and we affect it. Your mind-set affects your immune system, and your immune system affects your mind-set. Just as everything in the universe relates to everything else— everything within the body relates to everything else in the body. There has been a lot of research in the last twenty-five years exploring how the mind and body, and the body and mind, relate and communicate with each other, and a new science has developed called psychoneuroimmunology.

Psychoneuroimmunology is the study of the relationship among three systems: the nervous system (brain), the endocrine system (hormones), and the immune system (the protective system of spleen, thymus, lymph, and various cells). Pioneer-

175

ing research done by psychologists and scientists has come up with the confirmation that the mind does influence the state of health, and the state of health does influence the mind. This seemingly groundbreaking conclusion only confirms what you've probably observed in everyday experience: the depressed are more receptive to illness; a good mood makes you feel good all over.

▲

"In the classic experiments of the Russian physiologist Ivan Pavlov, dogs salivated when a bell rang because they had been trained so that their brains associated the sound with food. Now, American scientists have evoked a similar conditioned reflex to show that the brain can exercise direct control over cells of the immune defense system."
—HAROLD SCHMECK, *The New York Times*, January 1, 1985

▲

Research has established several key points about the mind-body relationship:

1. Mind-directed, cell-enhancing chemicals communicate directly with the immune system;
2. Mental attitude and mood can alter the course of disease;
3. The mind can "will" changes in the body;
4. Stress-related hormones weaken the immune system; and
5. Chemicals made by the immune system communicate with the brain. Basically, the brain "talks" to the immune system, and the immune system "talks" to the brain in an ongoing conversation.

Up until the 1970s it was assumed that the body and the immune system each lived lives of their own. With the discovery of the receptor site on an immune cell, and then the discovery of the neuropeptides with a special design to fit the receptor site, a breakthrough emerged. It became clear that communication from the brain to the body is not one-way. Many systems communicate with many other systems; there is a feedback loop.

The neuropeptides are made in the limbic-hypothalamus area of the brain, and they are also made in the stomach and elsewhere. They are a healing network throughout the body. Many dozens of neuropeptides have been identified, and they all have their own type of receptor. Imagine a lock and key; the receptor is the lock; the neuropeptide is the key designed to fit that lock. In this way, neuropeptides originating in the brain can talk to the spleen, or the liver, or the stomach, and neuropeptides originating in the spleen or liver or stomach can talk to the brain. It is an interrelated, mutually dependent feedback system.

▲

"Our emotional state will effect whether we'll get sick from the same dose of a virus."
—CANDACE PERT, Ph.D., *Journal of Immunology*, 1985

▲

Among the brain chemicals, discovered in the mid-1970s is a group referred to as endorphins; a contraction of the words "endogenous," meaning internal, and "morphine." The endorphins have a morphinelike effect—they dampen pain and increase good mood and positive mind. According to Dr. Bernard Bihari, endorphins are the most important systemic hormones involved in immune system functioning.

Endorphin receptors are found in the brain, spinal cord, digestive system, pancreas, spleen, kidneys, heart, lungs, reproductive organs, and the immune system. There is a receptor site for endorphins on the T cell of the immune system. If you visualize this T cell with a little spot like a dock, where the endorphin "lands," and imagine the endorphin energizes the T cell, so that it is more productive and does its job better— you will understand what an amazing discovery this is. We have chemicals in our body that can improve our health. How do we generate these chemicals? The body produces endorphins in response to laughter, music, beauty, exercise, smiling, happiness—and in general, all good, positive feelings.

From this knowledge, new to us in the last twenty years, it is clear that you can have a direct influence on your immune system. You are assured that you can take a role in determining your body status.

▲

"From a broader perspective, the neuropeptide system also may be the psychological basis of the folk, shamanistic and spiritual forms of healing currently returning to vogue under the banner of 'holistic medicine.' "
—Dr. Ernest Rossi, *The Psychobiology of Mind-Body Healing*, 1987

▲

Mind power is an often forgotten healing mechanism among holistic practitioners who are immersed in their own version of modern medicine—the illness and cure paradigm. Albert Einstein recognized an energy beyond the material. Physics now understands that matter and energy are convertible, and that the observer can affect the observed. It also assumes unity rather than separation. These new studies in consciousness confirm the ancients' understanding that humans are a whole unit of body, mind, and spirit. In ancient India the healing energy was called "prana," the Japanese called it

THE CIRCLE OF LIFE

**Brain
Releases
Chemicals
(i.e. endorphins)**

**Feeling
Wellness**

**Receptor
Sites on
Immune
Cells**

**Improved
Body State,
Strengthened
Immunity**

"ki," Polynesians, "mana," American Indians "orenda," and Chinese, "chi." Chi is referred to in the *Nei Chang*, the oldest book on medicine, as "an essential primordial energy that gives birth to all elements and is integrated into them."

NEW MIND-BODY RESEARCH

Since George Solomon coined the word "psychoneuroim-munology" (to reflect the relationship between the brain, the endocrine, and immune system) in 1964, much research has supported the mind-body connection, helped us understand how it works, and pointed the way to tapping into it. In the last twenty years:

- Research (1981) found that mice subjected to stress were less able to inhibit the growth of transplanted tumors.
- A study published in *Science* (Vol. 209, July 1980) concluded that "Emotional stress can lead to disease. The new field of behavioral medicine, first discussed at a Yale University conference in 1977, is based on an approach to disease treating mind and body as continuously interrelated. . . . Out of this developed the awareness that if we can control stress we can alter our susceptibility."
- Various research projects observe stress's power to weaken the immune system. One study correlated life stress events with illness seven to twelve months later. Another found the stress of an exam to college students caused a depressed immune system. "Stress is inextricably involved with the onset and prognosis for many diseases" (*Habits of Nervous Tension: Clues to the Human Condition*, C. B. Thomas, 1977).
- In a study reported in the *New England Journal of Medicine*, 1991, those who were exposed to a cold virus and who were highly stressed were five times more likely than low-stress subjects to become infected.
- A report in the *American Journal of Psychiatry* (143:1988) showed a correlation between psychological health and higher levels of certain immune cells.

- People who have good coping skills have the best immune response.
- Chronic emotional stress may be a "co-carcinogen"—so reported *Clinical Psychiatry News* (5[12]:40, 1978).
- Bereavement depresses the immune system.
- There is a learned immune response. Scientists found that mice with a weakened immune system could learn to override it.
- Nerve cells from the brain travel to the thymus gland (a key coordinator of strong immunity), and the thymus gland has nerve cells that travel back to the brain.
- Relaxation and meditation have reduced the need of diabetic patients for insulin.
- Immune cells directly influence cells in the brain, and Swiss researchers propose the idea of "immuneotransmitters."
- Positive attitudes may improve functioning.
- Unrelieved moderate to severe pain causes stress, which interferes with healing.
- There is evidence of a connection between hostility and heart disease and hostile persons are five times more likely to have a heart attack.
- There is documented evidence of spontaneous remission of cancer patients.
- Since there is spontaneous remission some people posited and then proved spontaneous prevention.
- Various therapies, including relaxation techniques, counseling, meditation, and yoga, have been found to manage stress and alleviate ailments, including arthritis, heart disease, gastrointestinal disorders, hypertension, and skin problems.
- Depression plays a role in immune suppression.
- The brain can learn how to regulate immune response.
- The power of suggestion is demonstrated by the placebo effect by which patients may find relief by just *thinking* that

they are taking a medication that is supposed to help them but which actually contains no medicine.
- Laughter produces measurable biochemical changes.
- Guided imagery can produce significant changes in the white blood cell count and enhance immunity.
- Candace Pert, noted brain researcher, wrote in the 1985 *Journal of Immunology*: ''A major conceptual shift in neuroscience has been wrought by the realization that brain function is modulated by numerous chemicals in addition to classical neurotransmitters.''
- In 1969 George Solomon reported that stress suppressed the immune system in animals.

▲

''It is relevant to note here that the psychological consequences of such stress mediated events have significant adverse effects on important elements of the immunological apparatus.''
—VERNON RILEY, ''Psychoneuroendocrine Influences on Immuno-Competence and Neoplasia,'' *Science*, Vol. 212, June 1981

▲

STRESS

Stress was defined in 1936 by Hans Selye as a nonspecific response by the body to any demand made on it to readjust. Stress can cause damage to body organs, the nervous system, and the immune system. Stress causes the release of hormones, adrenaline, noradrenaline, cortisol, and others. They are designed by nature to prepare a person for the fight-or-flight response: to provide an immediate reaction to an immediate danger. To achieve this they accelerate physiological responses—the blood pressure, heart rate, and blood sugar level increase and the blood clots more rapidly. The by-product of these body stress chemicals is the production of free radicals.

The stress reaction may also cause the movement of fat from body fat stores for use as fuel. This release of fat can also cause the release of fat-stored toxins, resulting in an increase of free radicals. When the practical response to stress that would have been helpful in fighting or fleeing from a wild animal, for example, which was what it was designed for, becomes instead chronic and continuing, it results in suppressed immunity and excess free radical production. In this case the intended benefits of the stress response become debilitating, with a loss of youthfulness, and the onset of early aging and disease.

Stress has many specific effects, including depletion of vitamins B_6 and C; deterioration of thymus, spleen, lymph nodes, liver, and other glands; weakening of T cell production; decreasing the number of lymphocytes; and depression of antibody synthesis.

An immune system weakened by stress leaves a body susceptible to infections and allergies. It can also lead to an increased heart rate, elevated cholesterol levels, muscle tension, and shortness of breath. Of course, a weak immune system is a factor in all disease.

Stress is caused by many and varied things, including being sick, having surgery, experiencing pain, fever, exposure to extreme heat or cold, overcrowding, noise, pollution, apprehension, fear, anxiety, and various emotional conditions.

▲

"It don't mean a thing if it ain't got that swing."
—DUKE ELLINGTON

▲

Add Up These Stressors to Learn Your Stress Level

EVENT	NUMBER VALUE
death of a spouse	100
divorce	73
marital separation	65
jail term	63
death of a close family member	63
personal injury or illness	53
marriage	50
fired from work	47
marital reconciliation	45
retirement	45
change in family member's health	44
pregnancy	40
sex difficulties	39
addition to family	39
business readjustment	39
change in financial status	38
death of a close friend	37
change in work	36
change in number of marital disagreements	35
mortgage payments or loan	31
change in work responsibilities	29
son or daughter leaving home	29
trouble with in-laws	29
outstanding personal achievement	28
change in living conditions	25
change in residence	20
other changes	15–20
vacation	13
Christmas season	12
minor violation of the law	11

▲

"Your problems, your moodiness, and many of your other problems come from the fact that you don't take death seriously. You think you live forever. If you knew that this is just a short time that's given to you, you'd probably appreciate it and use it better."
—Don Juan, *A Separate Reality*, by CARLOS CASTANEDA

▲

The Holmes-Rahe Social Readjustment Rating Scale

According to Holmes-Rahe, any score over 300 in a year's time would suggest a person had a high probability (they say 80 percent) of becoming sick. Of course, there are many other stressors, but the list on the previous page gives you an idea.

Keep in mind, the key to all this is how you react to the stress. It is not the stress itself, but your interpretation and response to it ("The Social Readjustment Rating Scale," T. H. Holmes, R. H. Rahe, *Journal of Psychosomatic Research*, 11, 1965, p. 216).

How Many of These Stress Reactions Do You Experience?

Always focusing on problems, in a "bad mood."
Difficult to concentrate, more disorganized than usual.
Feelings of unreality, weakness, "spaced out."
Overwhelming fatigue (this is also a symptom of a physical disorder, which is influenced by stress, or further aggravated by stress).

Difficulty sleeping, insomnia, wake up too early.
Having no appetite, or too much appetite—unusual weight
    gain or loss.
Inappropriate neurotic behavior, behavior out of your norm.
Trembling, sweating, fast heartbeat.
Generalized anxiety, for no special reason.
Behaving impulsively, not making sense for your best
    interests.
Procrastination.

THE EFFECTS OF STRESS

Stress

Adrenal glands activated
They release cortisone

Preparation for fight-or-flight syndrome
Sugar goes into the bloodstream
Protein released from organ storage

Thymus shrivels
Other organs depleted, pancreas, spleen, liver, and others
Nutrient reserves used up (especially vitamins B_6 and C)

Inadequate nutrients to replace those lost
Acid-alkaline imbalance causes acidity, which predisposes
to disease

When combined with

Constant continuing stress
Stress of pollution
Inadequate nutrients

Results in

Free radical production
Weakened immunity
Loss of youthfulness
Susceptibility to disease

Fight or Flight

The ancient response built into humans, the fight-or-flight response, is produced when you are confronted with a threat, a danger, or a fear. The body prepares to either fight, or to run away, and many hormones are released to help the body adjust quickly. Imagine a predatory animal on your path in early times. You would have had to mobilize all your power and energy to fight it, or to run as fast as possible. Either way, you need a quick input of glucose (sugars) into the bloodstream for energy, and to call up all reserves. The difference today is that it is not one or two stresses or confrontations per day, it is often almost constant. And it is this fact that is the key to the health damage of stress. The problem comes when the fight-or-flight response is continuing, when we are continuously under threat. The stress hormones that are released become constant and result in wearing down the body.

Selye pointed out something interesting: there is a good use for stress. Stress that is seen as positive can be challenging and encourage production of endorphins. He called this beneficial stress "eustress," like the word "euphoria." For instance, a child falling down as he learns to walk may be thought of as experiencing stress, but actually learning to walk may be so thrilling that the challenge brings on a sort of euphoria. All life's challenges may be seen in the same light.

Do Your Personality Characteristics Fortify Your Immune Function?

Some Questions:
Do I have a sense of meaningfulness in my work?
Do I have a sense of meaningfulness in my relationships?
Can I express anger when appropriate?
Am I able to ask for help and support when needed?
Am I able to ask for favors when needed?
Can I say no when I want to?
Am I self-determining in my decisions about my health-related behaviors—i.e., diet, exercise, etc.—or do I follow what I have been told without scrutinizing it?
Do I allow time for play and fun?
Do I let times of depression linger?
Do I indulge in thoughts that my life, or life problems, are impossible to change or improve?

Do I follow what is perceived as my duty in preference to
what I truly wish—i.e., fulfilling a role as parent,
friend, spouse—to the detriment of my own needs?

The above questions are adapted from the work of Dr. George
Solomon, considered the father of psychoneuroimmunology.

PROMOTING MIND-BODY HEALING

Tap into your own mind-body healing and health potential
by countering stress and stimulating endorphins. Counter stress
by exercising, deep breathing, staying optimistic, and choosing
pleasant work, companions, and environments. Stimulate endorphins through self-hypnosis, relaxation techniques, visualization, meditation, walking, and aroma therapy (discussed
later in this chapter).

▲

"The basic difference between an ordinary
man and a warrior is that a warrior takes
everything as a challenge, while an ordinary
man takes everything either as a blessing or a
curse."
—Don Juan, *A Separate Reality*,
by Carlos Castaneda

▲

Coping

The first step to managing stress is cutting it off at the
pass. See problems as challenges. Evaluate and explore what
you can do with the challenge. Write in your notebook, and
create a mental picture of the best outcome. At appropriate
time, take action.

Unresolved resentment and anger hurts *you*. Clear them out to pave the way for the endorphin flow, which will increase your vitality and make it easier to cope. This better coping will help reduce the problem and allow the feedback loop of mind–body, body–mind to flow.

▲

"They will build for me a temple and I will dwell within them."
—Old Testament

▲

"Whoever knows himself knows God."
—MUHAMMAD

▲

"The kingdom of God is within you."
—JESUS

▲

"May peace and peace and peace be everywhere."
—The Upanishads

▲

Laughter

Early healers understood the value of joyfulness and good humor in healing. The Old Testament pointed out: "A merry heart doeth good like medicine" (Proverbs 17:22). This splendidly sensible point of view held sway until the other religious philosophies took hold and the restrictions of polite behavior were imposed. About the same time, medicine developed the symptom and cure mode of healing, and the person's mood and environment as factors in well-being were set aside.

▲

"He deserves Paradise who makes his
companions laugh."
—MUHAMMAD, the Koran

▲

Luckily, when Norman Cousins, the former editor of the *Saturday Review* and then adjunct professor at the UCLA School of Medicine, got sick with a collagen disease with a fatal prognosis, inspiration struck. He decided to leave the hospital, stop taking medicine, start taking vitamin C, and watch funny movies. The Marx Brothers and Charlie Chaplin helped him to laugh himself well! He wrote a wonderful book documenting this, *Anatomy of an Illness* (Norton, 1979), in which he exclaims: "I made the joyous discovery that ten minutes of genuine belly laughter had an anaesthetic effect and would give me at least two hours of pain-free sleep." He returned to the subject in *Head First*, where he summarized the finding of Dr. Lee Burk at the Loma Linda Medical Center. He and his colleagues "measured changes in several 'stress' hormones in ten healthy male subjects after they viewed a sixty-minute humorous film. He found a significant increase in spontaneous immune cell proliferation accompanied by a marked decrease in cortisol, a hormone that has an immune suppressing capability."

Recent research documents that laughter decreases levels of the stress hormones. Laughter offsets the limitations of these immune weakeners, with the result that your immune system maintains its natural potential. This, combined with the immune-enhancing effect of your body's own opiates, the endorphins, puts you way ahead on the path of health. Maintain a good mood and you can profit from the healing power of laughter. Laughter stabilizes blood pressure, improves circulation, benefits digestion, oxygenates the blood, causes relaxation, and generally takes your mind off things, especially problems. The increase in endorphins and the decreased level of stress hormones combine for a healthier, stronger immune system that can efficiently counter free radical production.

BREATHING

As Steven Locke points out: "It is not stress itself which is immunosuppressive, but stress coupled with poor coping." What follows are some excellent coping techniques for stress relief.

In addition to the breathing exercises in the previous chapter, deep breathing, or what I call mindful breathing, is an excellent way to combat stress. Mindful breathing oxygenates the blood, eliminates waste, reduces anxiety and stress, and generally increases vitality.

In deep breathing you take in about seven times more oxygen as in a normal breath. When you retain the breath you send more oxygen to the bloodstream. Viruses and bacteria cannot live in a high oxygen environment. It is beneficial to deepen the breath through abdominal breathing, and to slow the breathing rate. Breath retraining has helped mitigate anxiety disorders, asthma, hypertension, and pain. The normal breathing rate is about sixteen to twenty breaths per minute. A health-building rate is about eight to twelve breaths per minute, and is characteristic of a calm, relaxed state. Deep breathing regulates the nervous system and counteracts stress.

Three Breathing Practices

COUNT YOUR BREATH

inhale to a count of 4

retain the breath to a count of 4

exhale to a count of 8

Sit comfortably. Set aside a few minutes, or more. Breath deeply to your abdomen. Close your eyes and count the numbers, 1 to 4, as you inhale. Hold the breath to a count of 4. Then smoothly exhale to a count of 8. Keep the counting smooth and the breath even. Continue. Empty the mind—when thoughts enter let them go and return to the count of the breath.

THREE-PART BREATH

inhale to a count of 6

retain to a count of 6

exhale to a count of 12

The 3 parts in the Three-Part Breath are the abdomen, the ribs, and the upper chest. Inhale to the abdomen, then continue the inhale to the ribs, let them expand to the side, then finish the inhale to the upper chest. Start the count 1, 2 to the abdomen, 3, 4 to the ribs, then 5, 6 to the upper chest. This way you get a complete breath. Hold the breath for a count of 6. Then exhale, starting from the upper chest 1, 2, then to the ribs 3, 4, then on 5, 6 exhale from the abdomen, finally bringing the stomach in toward the back. Relax and start the inhale again. Continue 10 rounds. Do more as you are accustomed to it. Be sure to keep the attention on the breath. If the mind wanders, as it will, let the thought go, and bring the attention back to the breath.

▲

"It is becoming increasingly clear that the human mind and physical universe do not exist independently."
—Edgar D. Mitchell, astronaut

▲

BELLOWS BREATHING
This is a form of yoga breathing that cleanses and energizes. Start by sitting comfortably, on a chair or on the floor with the legs crossed. Here, the exhale is emphasized. Start with the exhale. Forcibly contract the abdomen, sort of like a bellows. The breath will be exhaled. Then relax the abdomen and let the inhale happen. Follow immediately with a contraction of the abdomen and the exhale. In this breathing the chest does not move. It is the abdomen contraction that squeezes out the breath.

Do a round of 40 exhalations. Relax a moment, then inhale and hold the breath for a count of 16, letting the consciousness focus behind your closed eyes in the center of your forehead. Exhale and relax a moment. Repeat another round of 40 exhalations, followed by a long retention of a count of 16. Two rounds is fine to start with and you can build up later.

▲

"Assuming that you are normally constituted, there is no innate reason why you cannot heal any disease with awareness."
—DEEPAK CHOPRA, *Quantum Healing*

▲

MEDITATION

Benefits of Meditation
Muscle relaxation
Decrease in biochemical indicators of stress
Spiritual attunement
Increased intuition
Reduced metabolic rate—less oxygen consumed
Modified heart rate and blood pressure
Brain waves slowed—produces synchronous alpha waves (8 to 13 cycles per second)
Physiological age is reduced—for example, meditators in their fifties measured 12 years younger than controls on scales of physical aging

Three Meditation Practices

Meditate by Observing Your Thoughts
Meditation is a mental exercise aimed at calming the mind. Actually the process itself of meditating is the goal. By either focusing your mind on one thing—for instance looking at a flower, and just thinking about the flower, or saying a word and just thinking about the word—you allow your mind to rest, to let the chatter settle down. To get in touch with yourself, to observe your mind and its workings and to calm your mind, you can simply focus on your thoughts.

To do this: most importantly, choose a place, quiet, no disturbance. Set aside a time ten minutes, fifteen minutes. Do consistently. Daily. Sit and breathe smoothly and steadily. Whatever thought enters your mind, look at it for several seconds, then put it into a bubble, something like a balloon, and set it off to float away. The next thought do the same. Don't struggle to get rid of the thoughts, just allow them to enter, observe them, and then put the thought into the bubble and let it go. At first you may be flooded with thoughts. You may be surprised at the thoughts that pass through your mind that ordinarily you do not even notice. This awareness helps to settle the mind, and to bring an understanding of the "business" of the mind, and an acknowledgment that we can let some thoughts go, and cultivate others.

▲

"Meditation is a way of looking deeply into the chatter of the mind and body and becoming more aware of its patterns. By observing it, you free yourself from it."
—JOB KABAT-ZINN, in an interview in *Healing and the Mind*

▲

"Numerous studies in meditation conducted over the past decade have repeatedly shown that when a certain number of people enter into a particular state of consciousness, the world around them quite simply changes for the better."
—LARRY DOSSEY, M.D., *Space, Time and Medicine*

▲

Meditate by Counting Your Breath

Do the Count Your Breath breathing exercise—with a conscious attention to the count—inhale 4, retain 4, exhale 4. As you exhale, and as you inhale, keep your thought just on the count and the breath. When other thoughts enter—and they will—look at them, recognize them, and let them go. Return to the count. Before you start, set a time—five minutes perhaps to start and stay with it for that time.

Meditate on a Word

Another way of holding the attention is by repeating a word to yourself in your mind and keeping the attention on that word, or words. You could choose

All Is One
The God Within
Nature Heals

Sit in your chosen quiet place. Settle yourself for the time you have decided on—five to ten minutes. Choose your words, and repeat them to yourself; when other thoughts appear, look at them and let them go.

▲

"Close your eyes and you will see clearly.
Cease to listen and you will hear truth."
—Taoist poem

▲

Mindful Walking Meditation

Practicing mindfulness helps to reduce stress. Mindfulness is placing your attention in the present, being aware of what you are doing in the moment. A fine way of combining mindfulness with exercise and oxygen and full-spectrum light (see next chapter) is the Mindful Walking Meditation. According to Thich Nhat Hanh: ''The purpose of walking meditation is to be in the present moment and, aware of our breathing and our walking, to enjoy each step. Therefore we have to shake off all worries and anxieties, not thinking of the future, not thinking of the past, just enjoying the present moment.''

This is done by walking with conscious awareness. For instance, choose a pleasant place to walk with a specific distance that suits the time you can allow. Put the mind on the steps you take, the foot lifting, the foot going on the ground, the weight shifting, the breath inhaling and exhaling along with the pace of the steps. You may inhale on three steps and exhale on three steps, or four steps may suit you. Just what is comfortable. Be aware of your foot contacting the earth. If you are near trees, breathe in their oxygen, and breathe out your carbon dioxide. Breathe in the air-energy, breathe out toxins and stress.

Can you find twenty minutes to do this mindful walking every day?

Mind-Focusing Exercises

Magic Potion

Empower your hands by holding them 4 inches apart and circling them 3 times to the right over your head and 3 times to the left. Then sit in front of a table with a glass of pure water on the table in front of you. This water represents what you need—name it—it may be a potion for sleep, a potion to relax, a potion for energy, a potion to concentrate to do your writing, or painting, a potion for love, whatever. Place your hands surrounding the glass but not touching it. Magnetize the water, imaging the potion of your wish. Spend 1 minute in focused concentration, then slowly and very consciously drink the water, savor it, feel that it is the potion you need.

Do this first thing in the morning *before* talking to anyone. Continue for 13 days. Talk to your inner divine self, ask for help to potentize this water, spend 2 minutes, then totally center yourself and drink it slowly.

Crystal Liquid Detox

Take off your shoes and socks. Sit in a chair. Imagine that your feet are in a shallow pool of crystal water. Breathe in to a count of 3, hold breath for 3 counts, then exhale for 6 counts. Do this 3 times. Put hands palm up on your knees. Imagine your feet in a large pool of sparkling crystal water, surrounded by the softest tropical evening air. Tell yourself you are going to inhale through your feet and the water will come into your body washing over every cell, bathing and cleansing and picking up all toxins. As you exhale through your feet all toxins will go out into the pool water.

Prepare yourself and then do this: Inhale the crystal water through your feet, hold your breath to a count of 3 while imagining it reaching and cleansing every cell, then exhale to a count of 6 and watch the toxins go out through the feet into the pool of water as a gray stream that muddies the water as it goes out. Do this 3 times.

Sit quietly, a minute passes, and the crystal water turns clear again. Do this in the evening in the same way you brush your teeth—make it a habit.

▲

"Our consciousness is a field of all
possibilities. Anything is possible."
—DEEPAK CHOPRA, *Magical Thinking*, 1992

▲

Half a Day of Mindfulness

Take a half a day and spend it alone. Do everything slower and more attentively. Do simple projects like arranging books, or organizing the closet. Move about three times slower than usual.

Then go for a walk, and breathe as you count the steps. Then prepare something to eat. Chew each mouthful 20 times. Stay in the moment. That is the practice.

Send a Smile to the Thymus

The thymus gland is in the middle of your chest just below the collarbone. It produces important cells for the immune system. You can energize it by sending a smile. Start by feeling a smile. Imagine a smile. Now send this radiance in your imagination to the thymus, surrounding it with radiant smile energy. Hold this for 10 seconds and release. Know that your thymus is functioning better.

▲

"To obtain the inestimable benefits of meditation, you should first make a firm decision to practice every day. Your meditation room should be clean and quiet. Wear loose clothing and remove your shoes. Sit on a cushion, with legs crossed, in as comfortable a manner as possible. Keep your back straight. Your ears should be in line with your shoulders. Keep your tongue at the roof of your mouth and close your lips. Your eyes should be slightly open, unfocused on the floor

at a forty-five degree angle. Breathe through
your nostrils.

Hold your body erect, allowing breathing to be
normal. Many thoughts will crowd into your
mind. Let your thoughts come and go, without
getting involved in them or trying to suppress
them.

In your meditation, you yourself are the mirror
reflecting the solution of your problems. The
human mind has absolute freedom within its
true nature. You can attain this freedom
intuitively. Don't work toward freedom; but
allow the work itself to be freedom.

Practice this meditation in the morning or in
the evening or at any leisure time during the
day. You will soon realize that your mental
burdens are dropping away one by one, and
that you are gaining an intuitive power
previously undreamed of.

Don't doubt the possibilities of meditation
because of the simplicity of its method. If you
can't find the truth right where you are, where
else do you think you will find it?

You will soon discover the treasure of wisdom,
which in turn you can share abundantly with
others, bringing them happiness and peace.''
—Zen Master Dogen (1200–1253)

▲

AROMATHERAPY

Smells can be therapeutic. Have you noticed the soothing feeling when you walk through a pine forest? The brightness and inspiration in a garden of mixed flowers? The calm you feel around blossoming lavender? Yes, it is true. The smell itself as it is inhaled is processed by the limbic system in the brain. The limbic system is the source of emotional reactions related to survival, fear, and the response to stress, as well as being a regulator of heart rate, respiration, and blood sugar levels. The limbic system communicates with other areas of the brain, including the pituitary gland, which in turn sends chemical messengers into the blood, thus affecting the body and emotional state.

Aromatherapy is the use of natural and aromatic plants to enhance physical, emotional, and spiritual well-being. Essential oils are the concentrated essence of the plant and could be referred to as the ''soul'' of the plant. They help us to tune into the energy of the plant, which can support us on many levels including physiological and psychological. By using scents daily it is possible to improve mood, confidence, communication, and creativity, and it also helps stimulate the production of endorphins. Aromas have an effect on the emotional state, and in turn can enhance the immune system and correct imbalances.

Aromatherapy can be used at home, at work, in your car, in your bath and body oils, and for meditation. It can be used in many ways, including as a diffuser (in candles, in bath and body oil, perfume, or by putting a few drops of essential oil on the pillow), which disperses a fine mist of micro-particles. Some essential oils that counter stress are neroli, marjoram, lavender, bergamot, tangerine, rose, and sandalwood.

Some Essential Oils

OIL	BENEFICIAL EFFECT
Jasmine	euphoric
Clary sage	uplifting
Lemon	refreshing
Rosemary	encourages inspiration and imagination
Peppermint	digestive aid
Pine	counters fatigue
Eucalyptus	refreshing and balancing
Chamomile	soothing
Sandalwood	aids reflection and centering
Spikenard	sedative
Basil	increases alertness
Cedarwood	better physical energy
Mugwort	enhances creativity
Rose	brightens communication

In the near future it may turn out that the mind is more powerful than any of our other free radical fighters. The next chapter discusses another emerging and valuable resource, light.

CHAPTER 7

Light—The Sunshine Nutrient

"For the rest of my life I want to reflect on what light is." — *Albert Einstein*

*L*ight has remarkable healing qualities. Every area of your mental and bodily status is influenced by sunlight. Light also has the power to weaken health through free radical formation and cell mutation. This is especially so when compounded with the high-fat and low-nutrient diet of the modern human. The current scare about the ozone breakdown and skin cancer has focused the public on the damaging aspects of sunshine, while ignoring its great health benefits. It is crucial to receive the health-enhancing qualities of sunlight and at the same time minimize its risks. This involves being careful about exposure, and also being careful about reducing dietary intake of fats and increasing the free-radical-fighting nutrients.

▲

"Exposure to the sun is highly necessary in persons whose health needs restoring."
—HERODOTUS

▲

Sunlight could be considered another nutrient for humans—just as it is for plants. We know very well that our bodies require food, water, and oxygen, but in modern times the awareness of the value of sunlight has reemerged only recently. Ancient man worshipped the sun. In Egypt the sun god was extolled in many forms. In Greece, Zeus was regarded as a sun god and the Greeks promoted heliotherapy (helio = sun). Prior to this time, Babylon, Phoenicia, and Sumeria all had solar deities. Ancient feasts were centered on the sun. A key festival was in the third week of December marking the end of the short days of winter. The early Christian church placed the birthdate of Christ as December 25 so as to coincide with this pagan solar festival and thus win allegiance. Church control was installed and instinctive adoration for the sun was submerged.

The eighteenth and nineteenth centuries brought a back-to-nature philosophy and with it sanitariums, "cures," and solar therapy. In the late nineteenth century rickets was correlated with lack of sunlight. In 1903 Niels Finsen won the Nobel Prize for treating tuberculosis of the skin with ultraviolet (UV) light. In the 1930s the ability of UV light to kill bacteria was discovered. In 1975, a Russian study showed that exposure to UV rays doubled the body's ability to counter infection. Unfortunately, all this was soon outshone by the power of antibiotics to kill bacteria, and light therapy took a back seat. In the 1980s there came acknowledgment of the clearly detrimental effects of antibiotics (except in dire emergency when they can be a life-saver) and so we can again go back to nature and rely on sunlight to build health.

▲

"Light is sweet, and it pleases the eyes to see
the sun."
—Ecclesiastes 11:7

▲

An impediment to the return to the use of nature's free gifts is the pharmaceutical industry. As an example, in the realm of treatment for high blood pressure the worldwide sales for antihypertensives were $1.5 billion in 1985 (*The Economist*, "Molecules and Market," Vol. 306, No. 7484, February 1987) while a dose of sunlight can lower blood pressure at no cost.

As I write this I am on the veranda of a house in Florida in the shade, yet receiving the sun's beneficial rays indirectly through eyes and skin. It is only recently that I have come to appreciate the value of the "sunshine vitamin" that most of us have taken for granted.

▲

"There is some evidence in the scientific literature that sunlight can increase the energy level in human cells."
—ZANE KIME, M.D., *Sunlight*, 1980

▲

HERE COMES THE SUN

The sun, 93 million miles from the earth, emits energy in the form of electromagnetic radiation. Sunlight comes to the earth as waves of energy particles (photons), which move through space at a great rate of speed. They are measured in a length called a nanometer (NM), which is one billionth of a meter. Of all these waves, only about 1 percent can be seen by the human eye. Other invisible waves reaching earth are ultraviolet and infrared. The three components of solar rays reaching earth are infrared, visible light, and ultraviolet.

Infrared provides the heat we feel while in the sunlight. The visible light provides various wavelengths with various

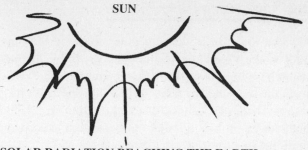

SUN

SOLAR RADIATION REACHING THE EARTH

Electric waves	Radio waves	Microwaves	Infrared	Visible light	Ultraviolet	X-rays	Gamma rays	Cosmic rays

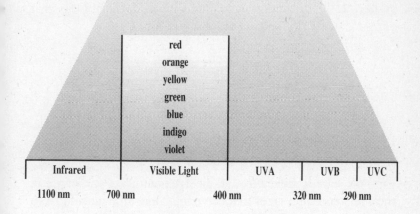

red
orange
yellow
green
blue
indigo
violet

Infrared	Visible Light	UVA	UVB	UVC

1100 nm   700 nm   400 nm   320 nm   290 nm

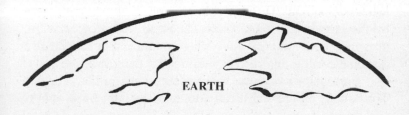

EARTH

biochemical effects that are determined by the absorption of particular wavelengths of light energy. In plants, for example, the chlorophyll in leaves looks green because it utilizes energy from the blue and red areas of the light spectrum for photosynthesis. The green light is reflected. In humans and animals, the hemoglobin in blood looks red because it absorbs green from the light spectrum.

Ultraviolet light is the part of the spectrum that has the most biological influence. It is, however, deflected by window panes and dark or regular glasses, thus blocking its benefits. Ultraviolet light comes in three bands, UVA, UVB, and UVC, depending on the wavelength. UVA causes light tanning, contributes to wrinkling, and nourishes the immune system. UVB causes sunburn, activates synthesis of vitamin D, can cause DNA damage and cell mutation, and can weaken the immune system. UVC is sometimes immune-suppressive, but it is also germicidal, so it kills bacteria and viruses.

▲

"We have finally learned that light is a nutrient much like food, and like food the wrong kind can make us ill and the right kind can keep us well."
—JOHN OTT, *Health and Light*, 1973

▲

We take in light through the eyes and the optic nerve in the eyes sends messages to the hypothalamus, the pineal gland, the pituitary gland, and other gland systems, depending on the spectrum of light. Through skin receptors, the melanin in the skin, responding to light, affects almost all physiological activities. The red blood cells in capillaries at the skin surface also respond to light, and convey messages to the rest of the body.

This chapter explores these connections further. The sun can enhance health and it can also do harm. This harm is now possibly increased with the breakdown of the ozone layer. The goal is to get the benefits without the damage.

▲

"Sunlight increases the use of oxygen in the
tissues. This can be very important in
stimulating the immune system especially in
the production of antibodies."
—ZANE KIME, M.D., *Sunlight*, 1980

▲

John Ott, a pioneer in the study of the effects of natural and artificial light on humans, came to his discovery serendipitously. He had been suffering from arthritis, and while in Florida working on his specialty of time-lapse photography of plants, he broke his glasses. He continued to work in the shade of a palm tree without the glasses. His arthritis got better, even to the point that X rays showed an improvement in the problem hip joint. Ott then began studying the effects of light on animals and humans and found that the key to receiving the full benefits light can provide is receiving light from the entire spectrum. He discovered in experiments with animals that they show a normal growth rate only when the full spectrum of light is present. In humans, many ailments are improved with sunlight, including high blood pressure, cancer, and chronic fatigue syndrome.

In 1973 Ott published his breakthrough study that shows how light influences you, *Health and Light*. This book tells how sunglasses may provoke illness, how indoor fluorescent lighting may bring on fatigue, hyperactivity in children, hypertension, and insomnia, and how full-spectrum indoor lighting can improve mood and health. Ott followed this book in 1982 with *Light Radiation and You* in which he concludes that full-spectrum light is the "missing link" in cancer research, and ties malignant melanoma to fluorescent lighting. Ott also describes several spontaneous remissions among cancer patients who removed themselves from artificial indoor lighting to outdoor sunlight.

▲

"Give me the splendid, silent sun with all its
beams full dazzling."
—WALT WHITMAN

▲

Additional research subsequent to Ott's work has continued that exposure to full-spectrum light is related to numerous health benefits. It increases the energy level in cells, acts as an antibacterial agent, enhances the body's resistance to infection, enhances oxygen transport to the blood, reduces cholesterol levels and blood pressure, balances blood sugar, has a relaxing effect, feeds the pineal gland, thereby enhancing immune integrity, causes synthesis of vitamin D in the skin, increases the white and red blood cell count, increases the total elevation of protein, augments liver function, offsets depression, stimulates the thyroid gland and thus helps weight loss, and stimulates enzymes.

▲

"There is more and more reason to think of
light as a kind of drug which, depending on
the situation and individual, can have good or
bad effects."
—"Light," *The New Yorker*,
January 14, 1985

▲

On the other hand, light can also be dangerous if you get too much exposure, or if your body is already stressed too much. It can cause production of free radicals, weaken the immune system, produce cataracts, age the skin, damage

DNA, and produce tumors and cancer if the immune system is already weakened and the diet is high in fat and low in nutrients.

FREE RADICAL FORMATION FROM SUNLIGHT

The process of free radical formation is accelerated by sunlight. The amount of fat in the diet is a variable that determines the extent of sunlight-caused free radical formation. Until recently humans had mostly olive oil and saturated animal fat as their source of fat. In the early twentieth century, they learned to extract oil from beans, corn, and seeds, and produced the much-touted polyunsaturated fats. Unfortunately, advertising promoted a false impression and many people switched from butter and olive oil with all their inherent nutrients to margarine, which is depleted of nutrients. Butter, for example, contains carotene, vitamin E, and minerals, while margarine has only added synthetic vitamins, if anything. At the same time, with sales of dairy foods, ice cream, and desserts booming, the average American consumed 35 to 40 percent of his calories in fats. This combination of polyunsaturated fats and increase in overall fat intake along with the loss of nutrients found in the whole fat resulted in increased free radical formation, weakened immunity, and early aging of skin.

▲

"Light enters the eyes not only to serve vision, but to go directly to the body's biological clock within the hypothalamus. The hypothalamus controls the nervous system and

endocrine system, whose combined effects
regulate all biological functions in humans.''
—JACOB LIBERMAN, M.D., *Light, Medicine
and the Future*, 1991

▲

According to much recent research on free radical formation, sunlight is only implicated as a culprit when the protective
free-radical-fighting nutrients are low. See Chapter 4 for more
information on supplements. So sunbathing, in moderation,
will either be of benefit or detrimental, depending on your
nutritional status. For a person with *in*adequate protective nutrients and a high-fat diet, sunbathing equals weakened immunity, aging of skin, and possible skin and other cancers. But
in a person with adequate protective nutrients and a low-fat
diet, moderate sunbathing equals strengthened immunity, increased sense of well-being, increased red blood cells, increased white blood cells, improved liver function (and so
better ability to deal with toxins), moderated blood pressure,
improved morale, and reduced likelihood of disease.

PINEAL GLAND

The pineal gland, located in the center of the head, re-
ceives light through the eyes, and it produces various chemicals. In particular it regulates the endorphins, the morphinelike
chemicals that, as we have seen, produce a good mood and
sense of well-being. Aside from this wonderful function, endorphins enhance the T cells of the immune system and in this
way counter the immune-weakening effect of free radicals.
The pineal gland also makes melatonin, which is stimulated
by the *absence* of light. Melatonin is made during the hours
of darkness and its sedative effect makes you drowsy and able

to sleep. It also slows general ability. So what, we may wonder, happens to twentieth-century people who are exposed to an additional four to seven hours of light due to electricity? Can we blame Edison for some modern health damage?

Melatonin has several health benefits in addition to its sedative effect. It has immune-stimulating qualities that slow the aging process. Research with animals showed an increase in longevity with melatonin over those deprived of melatonin. It has tumor-fighting properties and can slow the growth of some forms of cancer. In one interesting research project, rats were given leukemia cells; some were then given melatonin, and others not. Those with the melatonin developed fewer tumors. Melatonin is also found to reduce stress and control stress-related diseases. Once we consider the dependence we have on daylight and darkness, we will conclude that electric lights, which allow us to stay up at night, do not truly benefit us.

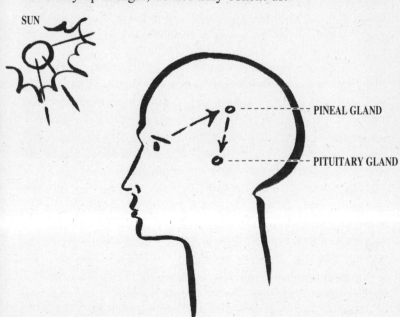

SUN

PINEAL GLAND

PITUITARY GLAND

▲

"The ozone layer, if it disappears, disappears
for all of us."
—ISAAC ASIMOV

▲

OZONE

The culprit in the sun's damage to the skin and immune
system is the production of free radicals. With the depletion
of the protective filtering layer of ozone around the earth, more
solar and cosmic rays reach our planet, causing excess free
radicals to be formed in the human body. We need, therefore,
to be more cautious in receiving the sun's splendid benefits,
because the guaranteed protection that once was there is now
vastly changed. Ozone has always been counted on to absorb
practically all the UVA and UVB radiation.

Ozone surrounds the earth in a layer between six and
thirty miles above sea level. It is formed when light rays strike
molecules of oxygen, which is O_2, and cause them to break
into two separate oxygen atoms, or O and O. An atom of
oxygen then combines with a molecule of oxygen and forms
ozone, which is O_3. Then ozone breaks down again as it absorbs the short light rays and recombines again.

In 1990, a severe ozone hole over Antarctica was de-
tected. In 1991, NASA data showed ozone depletion over the
Northern Hemisphere was occurring at a rate twice as fast as
predicted—200,000 additional cancer deaths were predicted
by the EPA as a direct result. A 1991 U.N. environment
program report on ozone depletion predicted millions of skin
cancer cases, cataracts, and disruption of food supplies and
ecosystems from the excess UVB radiation brought about by

ozone loss. In 1992 both NASA and the World Meteorological Society reported 10 to 25 percent ozone depletion measured over the northern United States and Canada, the Antarctica ozone hole being three times the size of the United States. There were reports in Chile and Argentina of a 200 percent increase in skin cancer since 1990. And in 1993, according to NASA, ozone levels in the first three months of 1993 were down 10 to 20 percent from their normal range in the middle latitudes of the Northern Hemisphere. Ozone depletion, and the attendant health problems, is a serious worldwide problem. As the ozone layer decreases, more and more of the sun's radiation reaches earth.

A 1 percent reduction in the ozone level is estimated to increase the amount of UVB reaching the earth by 2 percent. The Environmental Protection Agency estimates for every 1 percent decrease in the ozone layer the incidence of skin cancers will increase between 3 and 6 percent. Since 1960 there has been an increase in two forms of skin cancer, malignant melanoma and squamous cell skin cancer. Although researchers foresee a continuing increase in skin cancers and a weakening of the immune system due to the increase in UV rays we are now experiencing, this does not mean we should totally avoid light.

In spite of the fact that there are hundreds of articles in the medical journals telling about sunlight's great benefits to health, the prevailing refrain is a warning to stay out of the sun and to take precautions. This conflict is difficult to resolve. What emerges after scrutiny of the facts is moderation: to neither avoid sunlight completely, nor to bake in it. Strike a balance between some sun and too much sun.

John Ott points out: "Without doubt, too much UV is harmful. But the fear of getting too much ultraviolet is causing many people to overprotect themselves from sunlight, to the point they're creating a deficiency in a very essential life-supporting energy." In *Sunlight and Health*, Michael Lilly-quist writes: "Please note that even Ott does not suggest baking endlessly in the sun without protection. He typically advises sitting in the shade while receiving one's solar therapy. The idea is to be exposed, not overexposed, to all the wavelengths that reach the earth, none being artificially filtered by sunglasses, eyeglasses, or contact lenses."

Ott's views are confirmed by Jacob Liberman, an optometrist and author of *Light, Medicine and the Future*, who recommends sunning the eyes without sunglasses daily and using sunscreens sparingly.

▲

"Between eleven and three, slip under a tree."
—Old maxim

▲

THE EFFECT OF
UV RADIATION ON THE EYES

Of the three types of UV radiation, UVA is the most damaging because it is transmitted to the crystalline lens of the eye. But UVB, which is absorbed by the cornea, can also be harmful; it can cause snow blindness. UVC has so far been blocked by the ozone layer, but with further breakdown this could change.

The benefits of sunlight depend on light reaching the skin and eyes, the length of time exposed, and the amount of skin exposed. It is also affected by altitude, latitude, cloud cover (when it's overcast about 50 percent of UVB remains, for example), reflective surfaces (reflections from snow, sand, and water can double the amount of UV rays you receive), skin

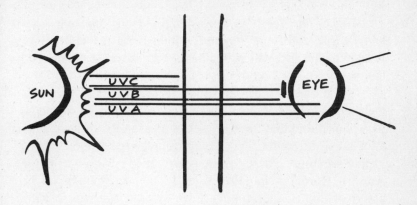

type, recent sun exposure (which would build up protection), the degree of ozone and filtering, and general sky light and indirect light, which transmits a lot of UV rays.

To reap the benefits and avoid the risks of sunlight exposure, avoid burning. Seek brief exposure, from fifteen to twenty minutes for light skin, up to forty minutes for darker skin, to build protection. Stay in indirect sun, on a porch for example, for several hours a day. John Ott recommends a "minimum of six hours a day of natural daylight." Remove contact lenses and glasses when appropriate. Use a hat to cut glare without blocking some of the beneficial UV rays. Avoid being out in the hottest hours, 10 A.M. to 3 P.M. Be aware if you are taking any photosensitizing drugs, as they increase UV effect. Some drugs can make you more sensitive to the effects of sunlight, including tranquilizers, diuretics, and antibiotics. Ten minutes of midday sun is all a body needs to synthesize the RDA of vitamin D, which is thought to have anticancer properties.

CHAKRAS

Light, like food, is nourishing. Among the many acknowledged nutrifying benefits of light is the fact that it provides vitamin D, which regulates the use of calcium and magnesium in the body.

Yet it has not been generally recognized that the colors themselves in the light benefit the body. Ancient Eastern teachings pointed out that there are seven areas in the body that are a focus for different colors, going from the red to violet of the visible spectrum. These locations are called chakras, from the Sanskrit word for spinning wheel. They are thought to be a sort of funnel, or stepping-down system, for transforming universal energy into physical energy.

Each chakra is anatomically related to an endocrine gland and to a part of the nervous system.

When the energy in a chakra is blocked or imbalanced it is believed to affect the related organ and the state of health. The ancients understood that the human energy field as focused in the chakras could be rebalanced with light. Among some

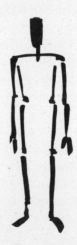

NAME	COLOR
Crown	Violet
Brow	Indigo
Throat	Blue
Heart	Green
Solar plexus	Yellow
Spleen	Orange
Root	Red

modern researchers who have delved into this aspect of light's benefits is Dr. Alexander Schauss of the American Institute of Biosocial Research in Tacoma, Washington, who believes that color is a form of energy that produces physiological changes. So, all the more reason to be outdoors and absorb the full-spectrum light of solar rays through your eyes and skin daily.

The Chakra System

GLAND	GOVERNS
Pineal	Relation with God
Pituitary	Relation to spiritual nature
Thyroid	Communication
Thymus	Center of love
Pancreas	Personal power
Adrenal	Survival
Sexual organs	Relationships, sex

SUNSCREENS AND SUNGLASSES

Yes, too much sun on the skin can be damaging, but too *little* sun exposure is also damaging. Sunscreens block the beneficial rays of the sun. A study published in 1988 in the *New England Journal of Medicine* showed that a group of men who worked outdoors without sunglasses had three times more cataracts than those who shielded their eyes. From this observation the conclusion was made that sunglasses are a must. However, remembering that there are other variables such as diet and level of nutrients, and also remembering that good health depends on absorbing some light through the eyes, a moderated balance is suggested: some light but not too much. There are full-spectrum eyeglasses—Eye Kraft Sun lite lens—ask for them at your eyeglass store. The best sunglasses are full-spectrum neutral gray manufactured by Keystone Optical Lab. Bausch & Lomb makes an ultraviolet transmitting contact lens called Soflens.

SEASONAL AFFECTIVE DISORDER, OR SAD

During the winter when there is less light, many people produce more melatonin and as a result develop a seasonal depression called SAD, or seasonal affective disorder, characterized by a lowering of energy, irritability, anxiety, or sleepiness. Windowless offices, dim lights, short days, and very little time outdoors—all add up to insufficient daylight, which can cause people to be in a dreary mood. To offset SAD, take a walk at midday, go out in the light daily without wearing glasses or contacts, or purchase a light box containing full-spectrum light and place it in your work area and spend a certain amount of time close to it daily. (See Part IV for sources of these lights.) It was found that several hours of artificial high-intensity full-spectrum light in the early morning brought about dramatic relief to people with SAD. Winter blues usually left within two weeks of starting light therapy. Dr. Damian Downing in his book *Daylight Robbery* recommends that SAD sufferers use a very bright light, at least 2,500 lux in intensity, to suppress melatonin production in the pineal gland. He recommends using the light as a source of illumination, but he also believes you should regularly spend time near it, basking in its light.

SAD Questionnaire

Researchers estimate that 10 million people suffer from SAD and about 25 million suffer from a lesser degree of this syndrome and experience "winter blues." If you answer yes to three or more of the following questions, you may be among them.

In the winter or early spring:

1. Do you have less energy than usual?
2. Do you feel depressed or sad for no discernible reason?
3. Do you need more sleep?
4. Do you have more food cravings, especially for carbohydrates?

ARTIFICIAL LIGHTING

Light is converted in the body to chemical energy, so when wavelengths are missing, as they are in artificial light, or filtered out of the spectrum of natural light by windows, windshields, or eyeglasses, a person is deprived of known benefits.

Not only are incandescent and fluorescent lights inferior to sunlight, they may actually be harmful to your health. There are many studies that have documented this, particularly those of John Ott. Possible harm from indoor lighting includes headache, eyestrain, nervousness, increased rate of tumor development (U.S. Bureau of Radiological Health), genetic mutation, and creation of cancer cells.

Research indicates that an improvement in the quality of artificial light is beneficial to health. For example, a study in a Vermont elementary school showed that the number of sick days was reduced 24 percent in the classrooms that used full-spectrum light (*Lancet*, November 21, 1987).

To improve indoor lighting, open the window for a "light bath," get special plastic UV-transmitting windows, get full-spectrum lenses for your glasses, and get a bank of lights for your work area and daily spend some time close to it.

Types of Indoor Lighting

Incandescent Bulbs

The usual sort of light bulbs. Most of their electricity is converted to heat and only about 10 percent goes into creating light. Their light causes eyestrain because only one part of the light spectrum is represented.

Full-Spectrum Incandescents

Usually called color-corrected and are more expensive than incandescent, but they last four times longer and have the full spectrum of visible light but no UV. They do not cause eye strain.

Halogen Lamps

Incandescents that have a cooler and brighter light and give more light per watt. They do not have the full spectrum of light.

Fluorescent Light

Connected to a host of health problems, including tumors, cancers, headaches, and nervousness, they are never a good choice, even the so-called daylight fluorescent.

Full-Spectrum Fluorescent Lights

Contain the full spectrum of light plus the UVA, which is known to help the body make vitamin D and also improves mood and productivity.

The Ott Light

John Ott developed a light system that contains full-spectrum tubes, a separate UV light, and grounding. It is electronically ballasted and so operates at 20,000 to 60,000 cycles per second and does not give off a disturbing electromagnetic field, as do other fluorescent bulbs.

Light Boxes

Used for treatment of SAD. A bank of three or four full-spectrum fluorescent bulbs is set in a box. It is recommended to put this near your work area and to sit near it for at least one or two hours a day, especially first thing in the morning.

Yes, light, mind power, stress avoidance, exercise, supplements, and foods are all avenues to countering the health-damaging excess free radicals we face today. The following chapter discusses pollution, which is a prime cause of these threatening excess free radicals, and thus the most important point of consideration.

CHAPTER 8

Pollution—Who Needs It?

"If they can get you asking the wrong questions,
they don't have to worry about the answers."
    —*Thomas Pynchon,* Gravity's Rainbow

*Y*our body is bombarded by pesticides and all kinds of hazardous chemicals. It is surrounded by man-made radiation, including the residue of the over 800 atmospheric atomic bomb tests up until 1963 as well as the health-damaging releases from the normal everyday operation of the world's 400 nuclear power plants and fallout from nuclear accidents. Two hundred twelve million pounds of hazardous waste is generated every day in the United States and more than 55,000 synthetic chemicals are now in regular production.

▲

"All that is necessary for the triumph of evil is
that good men do nothing."
—EDMUND BURKE

▲

A recent list of chemicals that are considered capable of causing cancer included 1,500 substances. Many of these are in our everyday environment—in medicines, food additives, and

224

directly in the food in the form of pesticides and the waste runoff from various industrial processes.

Exposure to pollution can cause excess free radical production. Some common sources of pollution are: heavy metals like lead, mercury, and copper, low-level radiation, radon, cigarette smoke, food irradiation, and impure or overly chemicalized tap water.

The effects of some of these toxins may not be apparent for years, making it difficult to connect cause and effect. The poor state of our national health—with, for just one example, cancer deaths rampant, going from one out of four in 1975 to a predicted one out of two in the year 2000 and a state of widespread degeneration becoming the norm—makes it increasingly apparent that these toxins are to blame. Of course, there are other factors to consider. One, for example, is our depleted soil and the food grown on it, which no longer has its intrinsic protective powers.

Toxins can damage the body in various ways, including free radical formation. They can enter the body and become systemic, damaging the liver and kidneys, the two organs of detoxification. They can reduce digestion of nutrients, alter and slow action of enzymes, block neurotransmissions, and even damage DNA.

▲

"Never doubt that a small group of thoughtful,
committed citizens can change the world.
Indeed, it's the only thing that ever has."
MARGARET MEAD

▲

Several variables determine what damage results from a person's exposure to toxins: genetic makeup, the amount of protective nutrients, the amount of toxins exposed to, the damage already done by other toxins, the amount of protective brain chemicals like endorphins, and the amount of beneficial sunlight and oxygen.

General planetary pollution, with its ramifications in the loss of trees, forests, and plankton, depletion of the protecting ozone, poisoning of air and water, loss of good topsoil, must all be dealt with at the source. With psychological work since Freud looking at the past, and then more recently focusing on the "inner child," it seems that a linear, cause-and-effect approach to mental health has resulted in a diversion of attention—a looking back, or inside—rather than a looking outward. Meanwhile, around us, the earth is being poisoned. Our life support system is sinking. *Look around!*

▲

"We have grasped the mystery of the atom,
and rejected the Sermon on the Mount."
—GENERAL OMAR BRADLEY

▲

We interrelate with the polluted state of our habitat by forming free radicals, which weaken our state of health. The question of the moment becomes: can we maintain a habitable planet? By changing your health status you will improve both your judgment and your energy, and your higher level body chemistry will cause a change on earth. The health of the Earth *depends* on your health by virtue of the influence you have, directly and indirectly, on critical decisions now being made. And by cleansing the earth you can, in turn, vastly increase your health potential.

YOUR HEALTH DEPENDS ON THE HEALTH OF THE EARTH

An article in the *New England Journal of Medicine* in 1981, "New Scientific Evidence and Public Health Imperatives," pointed out that research confirms "very low levels of toxins are capable of causing serious health effects.'' And goes on to suggest: ''Perhaps it is time to reexamine whether scientific standards of proof of causality—and waiting for the bodies to fall—ought not give way to more preventive public health policies.''

The Delaney Clause of the 1958 U.S. Food, Drug and Cosmetic Act prohibits the use of cancer-causing food additives in any amount. At the same time, however, the Delaney Clause allows the EPA to allow pesticide residues in foods. A 1988 amendment to the Delaney Clause called for a nine-year testing period of the 800 ingredients found in pesticides approved prior to 1988. The testing addresses cancer only. It does not address the effects of eating more than one pesticide at a time or the synergistic effect of the combination.

Toxic chemicals can attach and take electrons from molecules, thus weakening the immune system. They can cause cancer by attaching electrons in the DNA, thus creating a mutation.

▲

''No creature, not even swine, befouls its nest
with such abandon as does homo sapiens,
poisoning his habitat with fiendishly concocted
chemicals and their deadly toxic waste. A
morass of rotting human flesh awaits us all
unless the antidotes are rapidly applied.''
—CHRISTOPHER BIRD, *Secrets of the Soil*,
1989

▲

PESTICIDES

Concern over pesticides is increasing, and books listing what pesticides may be found in what foods are now available.

If all this is giving you heartburn, it is suggested that you choose organic foods. Why? Consider the deleterious health effects of pesticides: damage to the central nervous system; damage to the kidneys and liver, cancer; eye, nose, and throat irritation; chemical sensitivities; weakened immune system; depression; brain wave changes; psychosis; generalized complaints; headache; aching bones; fever seemingly due to flu or cold; and decreased brain alpha activity, which in turn weakens immunity.

Pesticides—insecticides, herbicides, rodenticides, and fungicides—are made to kill living organisms. Common sources of exposure are from foods, substances used to kill household pests, and those used on lawns and gardens.

▲

"The supreme reality of our time is the vulnerability of our planet."
—JOHN F. KENNEDY, 1962

▲

Facts Regarding Pesticides

- Pesticide use tripled from 1965 to 1985.
- In 1987 the National Academy of Science estimated that 90 percent of fungicides, 60 percent of herbicides, and 30 percent of insecticides pose a cancer risk to humans.
- In 1989 farmers used about 460 million pounds of pesticides on food crops.
- New imported foods come from countries with less strict regulation of toxins.
- In the 1930s there were 7 insects resistant to pesticides—in the 1980s there were 447 insects resistant to pesticides.
- The FDA tests only 1 percent of our food for pesticide residue.
- At least 17 percent of the 18 million children one to five

years of age are eating residues of toxic pesticides at unsafe levels.

- In 1990, U.S. manufacturing companies reported releasing 4.8 million pounds of toxic chemicals into the air, water, and ground.
- The National Academy of Science in 1987 reported that 90 percent of pesticides have not been adequately tested for their effect on health.
- The EPA states that 99 percent of the population has one or more toxic chemicals in their fatty tissues, many of which are linked to cancer.
- 95 percent of mother's milk is toxic.
- Depression, which can be caused by chemicals, affects one third of the population at some time of their lives.

Is it any wonder that sales of organic foods increased from $174 million to $1.25 billion between 1980 and 1989?

▲

"Our God isn't up in the clouds somewhere waiting for us to die. He's in the trees and the rocks and the four-leggeds."
—ROLLING THUNDER

▲

Since 80 percent of identified cancer risk comes from pesticides in fifteen foods, be cautious with:

Tomatoes	Beef
Potatoes	Oranges
Lettuce	Apples
Peaches	Pork
Wheat	Soybeans
Beans	Carrots
Chicken	Corn
Grapes	

CHEMICALS: DANGEROUS AT A DISTANCE

These very toxic chemicals manufactured in the United States are dangerous to a person 200 feet from a chemical leak:

CHEMICAL AND ITS USES	AMOUNT THAT IS DANGEROUS	U.S. PRODUCTION CAPACITY PER YEAR
Benzyl chloride: Perfumes, dyes, drugs, former war gas	1.4 lb	150 million lb
Chlorine: Bleach, water purifiers	2.5 lb	27.7 billion lb
Demeton: Insecticides	13 oz	N/A
Hydrofluoric acid: Metal cleaning, glass etching	9.5 oz	539 million lb
Hydrogen cyanide: Electroplating, photo processing	1.5 lb	1.3 billion lb
Formaldehyde: Fertilizers, dyes, resins, insulation, preservatives	3.5 lb	8.6 million lb
Methyl isocyanate: Pesticides	1.3 lb	12 million lb
Phosgene: Dyes, pesticides	6.5 oz	2.1 billion lb

Chemical and Its Uses	Amount That Is Dangerous	U.S. Production Capacity Per Year
Sulfuric acid: Dyes, glue, batteries, metals, explosives	2.5 lb	111 billion lb

—Environmental Protection Agency,
  SRI Directory of Chemical Producers,
  as quoted in *The New York Times*, December 17, 1985

▲

"Multiple Chemical Sensitivity (MCS) is an
illness in which patients experience adverse
health effects from low levels of
chemicals. . . . The influence of environmental
chemicals on mental health has been well
documented in the medical literature. For
instance pesticide exposure can cause
depression, anxiety, sleep disturbances or
psychosis."
—Cindy Dueiiring, "Depression and the
Chemical Connection," *Environment and
Health*, November 1992

▲

There are several steps you can take to protect yourself.
Buy produce that is certified organic (see chapter 3 for more
on organic food). Grow food in your own garden without
chemicals. If the vegetables you are eating are not organic,
wash them in a solution of one-half teaspoon dishwashing
liquid to a tub of water. Peel produce. Avoid foods from Latin
America, particularly Mexico and Chile, because of especially
high pesticide use there. Don't use chemicals around the house.
  There are many natural bug repellents you can use. For
roaches, use boric acid. To keep mosquitoes away increase

your intake of B vitamins and reduce intake of sugar and alcohol. Other ways of warding off mosquitoes are by rubbing garlic on your skin or by making an infusion of chamomile and rubbing it on your skin every twenty minutes.

Use alternatives to pesticides like insecticidal soap and organic pesticides. Encourage other predatory insects. Keep plants well fertilized and strong. Rotate crops.

▲

When asked what whites could learn from the Indian culture, Russell Means answered with one word: "Respect."

▲

TOXIC METALS

Toxic metals such as lead, mercury, aluminum, and cadmium are almost the norm now, so it is important to know that they cause free radical formation and weaken your immune system. They also tax the liver and the kidneys. Luckily, with a cleansing diet and supplements, you can eliminate them from your system.

To give you an idea of the implications of just one of these toxic metals, it is estimated that at least 38 million Americans have a significant level of lead in their bodies, a metal that can cause significant physiological and psychological impairments.

▲

"To have risked so much in our efforts to mold nature to our satisfaction and yet to have failed in achieving our goal would indeed be the final irony. Yet this, it seems, is our situation."
—RACHEL CARSON

▲

Toxin	Source	Potential Health Hazard	Antidote

Mercury	water-base paint
	pesticides
	"silver" fillings
	fertilizers
	some cosmetics
	floor wax,
	  plastics
	electrical
	  apparatus
	tuna and
	  swordfish
		allergies
		brain damage
		neurological
		  damage
		weakened
		  immune
		  system
			selenium
			detox diet
			vitamins A,
			  C, E
			Kyolic
			algae

Aluminum	buffered aspirin
	antacids
	baking powder
	pots and pans
	aluminum foil
	deodorants
		nerve and brain
		  cell damage
		hyperactivity in
		  children
		impaired thyroid
			zinc
			vitamin C
			Kyolic
			algae

Cadmium	cigarette smoke
	air pollution
	tap water
	fertilizers
		kidney damage
		loss of zinc
		weakened
		  immune
		  system
			zinc, vitamin C
			adequate fiber
			cabbage-family
			  vegetables
			Kyolic
			algae

Lead	car exhaust paint applied before 1978	brain damage kidney damage liver damage	calcium, zinc adequate fiber Kyolic

Toxin	Source	Potential Health Hazard	Antidote
Lead	ceramic glaze artist's paints solder insecticides lead water pipes	psychological problems	algae

Blood tests will indicate the circulating level of recent exposure to toxic metals. The hair test for toxic metals done by some health practitioners indicates levels over a period of time and so is a better guide.

"Typical of the subsidiary problems within the whole human survival problem is that of pollution in general—pollution of our air and water, but also of the information in our brains. We will soon have to rename our planet 'Poluto.' "
—R. Buckminster Fuller, *Operating Manual for Spaceship Earth*, 1969

▲

LOW-LEVEL RADIATION

The government-sponsored National Academy of Sciences stated in a report titled *Biological Effects of Radiation* (December 1989) that there is no safe level of radiation and this is because even the smallest amount causes free radicals. A number of independent researchers have demonstrated that long-term, relatively low levels of radiation may wreak up to 1,000 times more biological havoc than the currently accepted "risk levels" that are being used as reference points for decisions about licensing and operating nuclear plants.

In 1972, a researcher in Canada, Dr. Abram Petkau, found that when cells were irradiated slowly, a smaller total dose was needed to cause damage. Since this critical discovery it has been verified that a small dose of radiation over a long time is more damaging than one larger dose. Imagine the ramifications! This would mean that the small amounts of radiation that are released from the everyday operation of the world's 400 nuclear plants are doing much *more* damage than calculated.

▲

"Recent studies have suggested that free radicals can stimulate the activation (and proliferation) of HIV."
—C. Sappey et al. of the Grepo Laboratory in Grenoble, France, paper given at the VIII International Conference on AIDS, July 1992

▲

This discovery, known as the "Petkau Effect," showed that the amounts of radiation that are legally released from nuclear power plants, combined with the leaks, spills, and accidents, are a cause of extreme damage to our health because continuous low-level exposures produce hundreds to thousands of times more free radicals than the same dose delivered at one time, as in an X ray, for example.

Dr. Ernest Sternglass, a pioneering researcher in the field of radiation health, explains in his 1978 book *Secret Fallout* the implications of this new understanding: "Doses of radiation delivered slowly and continuously over extended periods of time are hundreds of times as damaging biologically as short, high intensity exposures of the same total dose. This was made clear in 1972 by Dr. Abram Petkau who discovered that at low doses of radiation absorbed at low rates, the dominant biological damage is produced by highly toxic molecules called free radicals.''

▲

''Nuclear power is life-threatening in three independent ways, each formidable. First, is the danger of accidents. Second, every nuclear reactor produces as a by-product plutonium-239, which is the most dangerous toxic substance known. Third, no one knows what to do with nuclear waste.''
—DR. GEORGE WALD, Nobel Laureate

▲

''Health effects from low-level radiation include the induction of cancer, genetically determined ill-health, developmental abnormalities, and some degenerative diseases.''
—Nuclear Regulatory Commission Report, December 1989

▲

The everyday releases of radioactivity by nuclear power plants has been found to cause several kinds of health damage, including premature births, congenital defects, infant mortality, mental retardation, heart ailments, arthritis, diabetes, allergies, asthma, cancer, genetic damage, and chronic fatigue syndrome. It has been linked to previously unknown infectious diseases, and generally weakens the immune system. Radiation shortens the life span of most organisms, according to Denham Harman in *Free Radical Theory of Aging*. Even at low levels, radiation may increase mutations of bacteria and viruses, as Andrei Sakharov described in his 1992 *Memoirs*.

A 1966 report by the Atomic Energy Commission produced findings that agree with the thoughts of Nobel Laureate Linus Pauling: "There are no safe amounts of radiation. Even small amounts do harm."

But humans evolved in an environment that contained naturally occurring radiation. So why is radiation so hazardous to us? The answer to this has to do with the *type* of radiation. Radon, which was always around (see below), is known as alpha radiation. The particles cannot travel very far. Strontium-90, which is a man-made radiation, is a beta particle. It *can* travel far. So how does this affect us? Our bones are hollow inside, they have a space for the bone marrow. This is the place where the white blood cells, which are key operatives in the immune system, are made. Nature did a brilliant design here because the bone protected the delicate bone marrow from the then-prevalent type of radiation—alpha. Nature did not foresee that humans would come up with a type of radiation that did not suit its original design. Because beta particles can travel through bone, they are able to zap the white blood cells. What happens? We gradually have a more and more weakened immune system. What is the answer to this dilemma? This seems to be the question confronting humanity.

HALF-LIFE OF RADIOACTIVE ELEMENTS

When a radioactive, or unstable, atom decays, it loses particles from its nucleus. The half-life of a radioactive substance is the time it takes for half of it to decay. The half-life can range from seconds to many thousands of years. During this time the substance is hazardous to life: plant, animal, and human. Multiplying its half-life by twenty gives a substance's full radioactive life. For example, the half-life of strontium-90 is 28 years. It will be stable, or not radioactive, in 560 years ($28 \times 20 = 560$). The chart below makes clear that our exposure to radiation is not only a critical issue now, but a long-term one as well—an unfortunate legacy to leave to future generations.

Substance	Half-life
Phosphorus-32	14.3 days
Phosphorus-33	25.0 days
Manganese-54	303.0 days
Iron-55	2.6 years
Iron-59	45.1 days
Cobalt-60	5.3 years
Nickel-63	92.0 years
Tungsten-185	75.8 years
Uranium-237	6.8 days
Xenon-133	5.3 days
Iodine-129	17 years
Iodine-131	8.1 days
Strontium-89	52.0 days
Strontium-90	28.1 days
Zirconium-95	65.0 days
Ruthenium-106	367.0 days
Tellurium-129m	34.0 days
Cesium-136	13.0 days
Cesium-137	30.2 years
Barium-140	12.8 days
Plutonium-239	24,400 years
Plutonium-240	6,850 years

▲

"In 1975 there were 59 cases of Lyme Disease recorded; in 1985, the number increased to 863, mainly in the two counties of Middlesex and New London, Ct., near the Millstone Nuclear Power Plant. Just as increases in cancer may be linked to the huge radiation release from Millstone in 1975, so too may be the tick-borne Lyme Disease epidemic. The Lyme Disease is carried by a spirochete that had not been harmful to humans prior to 1975. It is well known that radiation can cause mutations in bacteria. The enormous 1975 Millstone radiation release may have caused just such a mutation in the tick-borne spirochete.

—Jay Gould, Ph.D., *Deadly Deceit* (Four Walls Eight Windows, 1990)

▲

"Contrary to widespread belief, nuclear power is no longer a cheap energy source. In fact, when the still unknown costs of radioactive waste and spent nuclear fuel management, decommissioning and perpetual care are finally included in the rate base, nuclear power may prove to be much more expensive than conventional energy sources, and not economically competitive with safe, renewable resource energy alternatives such as solar power."

—*Nuclear Power Costs*, Report No. 95–1090, U.S. Government Printing Office, 1978

▲

Nuclear power emissions reach you directly in the air and water—and through animals we eat that may be contaminated with radiation, since they, in turn, consume air, water, and food that is contaminated. Radiation contaminates rainwater. We eat crops irrigated with this water. We inhale the air. Emissions may go to the land, into runoff, and then into rivers. Water may also find its way to a reservoir from which we drink. We eat fish from contaminated rivers and lakes. Freshwater fish are more contaminated than ocean fish because the minerals in the ocean water stop absorption of radionuclides to some extent. Fresh water contains 100 to 1,000 times the amount of strontium-90 that ocean water contains (C.S. Clusek, Department of Energy Lab Report, EML-429, July 1984).

Low-level radiation gets into the air and water through releases from nuclear power plants (planned and accidental), leaks from nuclear waste sites, nuclear military installations, nuclear bomb tests, medical procedures, tobacco smoke, air travel, smoke detectors, and X rays. See page 427 for resources to more information.

ENERGY CONSERVATION AND ALTERNATIVES

The transition from a nuclear- and fossil-fuel-based energy to a renewable form is both necessary and doable. With a fraction of the funds put into nuclear power we could readily tap the available sources of energy that are sustainable, reliable, and competitive—and are also clean and safe. These include wind power, hydroelectric power, tidal power, biomass (wood), geothermal energy, solar thermal technology, solar power, and solar cells. (Consider, for instance, that we could meet the world's demand for energy if the state of Nevada was covered with solar cells.)

Conservation of energy is also key. Each person can do

his part. Install double windows to conserve heat loss. Turn off the lights—half of electricity used for lighting is wasted. Use new refrigerators and other appliances that reduce energy consumption. Use new light bulbs that use one fourth of the energy. And these are just for starters.

▲

"We propose that energy efficiency, conservation, and self-renewing sources such as sun, wind, and water be implemented globally as an alternate to nuclear power and fossil fuels."
—A statement representing the wishes of all the world's women formulated at the Women's Congress in Miami, 1991

▲

The Rocky Mountain Institute in Colorado, a key advocate and resource for information on how to get away from reliance on destructive and polluting energy sources, estimates that replacing lighting, heating, and cooling systems along with design improvements in transmission lines could reduce U.S. electricity consumption by 75 percent. Many valuable groups are working to actualize the use of clean energy, and among them is the Union of Concerned Scientists, who have a nationwide "Renewables Are Ready" education campaign. See Part IV for resources on this critical topic.

▲

"No more than one or two decades remain before the chance to avert the threats we now confront will be lost and the prospects for humanity are immeasurably diminished. We, the undersigned senior members of the world's scientific community, hereby warn all of

humanity of what lies ahead. A great change in
our stewardship of the Earth is required.''
—*Warning to Humanity*, issued by the Union
of Concerned Scientists, 1992, signed by 1,500
scientists from 69 nations

▲

RADON

Radon is a radioactive gas that can be found in soils and
rocks that contain uranium, which is normally found in nature.
Radon is also found in soil that has been contaminated with
industrial waste, the by-products of uranium mining, or seepage from radioactive waste dumps, or perhaps from gases from
the underground bomb testing that went on from 1963 until the
1992 moratorium. Radon levels can vary to a great extent
depending on the construction of the building and how well
insulated it is. It is estimated that about 20 percent of American
homes have unacceptable levels of radon.

An insulated basement may not allow radon to ventilate.
Some rock structures contain a high level of radon; high levels
may even come from granite rock used to build a fireplace.
Well water in a high radon area may be contaminated, as may
be bath and shower water. The burning of coal releases radon,
as does seepage from underground nuclear bomb tests and
radiation waste dumps. To reduce the level of radon in your
home, use plenty of natural ventilation, as well as forced ventilation and cover exposed earth, seal cracks and openings.

▲

"The damage caused by ionizing radiation
results from free radical formation."
—Jane Brody, "Natural Chemicals Now
Called Major Cause of Disease," *New York
Times*, April 26, 1988

▲

Get the radon level in your home checked (see Part IV).
Here is how to interpret the results:

+   1.0 WL or higher; or 200 pCi/L or higher   About the
     highest reading observed in homes and deserves
     immediate attention, either by improved ventilation in
     the house or by relocation.
+   0.1 to 1.0 WL; or 20 to 200 pCi/L   Way above
     average, this amount is dangerous and warrants
     immediate attention. Equivalent to about 2,000 chest X
     rays per year.
+   0.02 to 0.1 WL; or 4 to 20 pCi/L   Above average.
     This amount would be equivalent to approximately 250
     chest X rays per year or two packs of cigarettes a day.
+   0.02 WL or lower; or 4 pCi/L or lower   Considered
     average but does carry some risk.

WL   = Working Level
pCi/L = picocurie per liter of air

SMOKING

Cigarette smoke, which is just another kind of pollution,
can cause formation of free radicals. It contains cadmium and
lead and a host of carcinogens, including benzene and formaldehyde. Cigarettes also contain radioactive polonium-210,

which causes free radical formation and ultimately could be responsible for immune suppression and cancer. The smoke from cigarettes contains carbon monoxide, which binds with hemoglobin in the red blood cells and makes it less able to transport oxygen around the body.

The Environmental Protection Agency declared second-hand cigarette smoke a Class A carcinogen, that is, one that causes cancer in humans. The EPA has designated only eight other Class A carcinogens, including asbestos, radon, benzene, and arsenic. The EPA report also concluded that secondhand smoke increases the severity of symptoms in up to 1 million children with asthma; causes approximately 3,000 annual lung cancer deaths in healthy nonsmokers; and increases the risk of developing asthma.

▲

"Children fed irradiated wheat developed polyploid cells and abnormal cells in increasing number (related to amount they ate). In contrast NONE of the children fed un-irradiated diet developed abnormal cells. Polyploid is associated with malignancy."
—J. BHASKARAM et al., "Effects of Feeding Irradiated Wheat to Malnourished Children," *American Journal of Clinical Nutrition*, February 1975, pp. 130–35

▲

FOOD IRRADIATION

Food irradiation is a process by which foods are exposed to a radioactive source, such as cobalt-60 or cesium-137, in order to extend the foods' shelf life by destroying some of the microorganisms that cause decay. Irradiation also controls ripening and sprouting. The radioactive material used is waste from nuclear plants. But the effects on health can be dangerous. In studies of animals, it was found that irradiated food caused tumors, kidney damage and chromosomal abnormalities, birth defects and liver disease. In studies of humans it was found to cause blood abnormalities. There have yet been no long-term human studies.

Free radicals are formed in the food by irradiation, and cancer-causing and mutation-causing chemicals, such as benzene and formaldehyde, are produced. Irradiation depletes the antioxidant vitamins A, C, and E and destroys some of the B vitamins, and alters proteins and fats. The microorganism that causes botulism is radiation-resistant, and may overgrow as other bacteria are knocked out, allowing them to grow without competition. Irradiation may cause carcinogenic molds to grow, and may cause mutations of some microorganisms.

Food irradiation also holds hazards for the health and safety of the general public. There is a possibility of accidents transporting these radioactive materials from the nuclear plant to the irradiating plant, as well as potential for workplace accidents. Disasters, natural and otherwise, like earthquakes, explosions, or fire, would be greatly exacerbated.

▲

"If the bacteria which produce the spoiled poultry's odor which hints at the presence of 'Clostridium botulinum' are killed and the botulism is not, consumers would die from their very first taste of Hiroshima hens. They just won't know whether or not the poultry is contaminated, because irradiating the food has removed nature's warnings."
—Dr. MORTON WALKER, in *The Townsend Letter for Doctors*, 1992

▲

History of Food Irradiation

- 1909: Franklin Smith of Philadelphia patents the use of X rays to kill beetles that feed on tobacco plants.
- World War II era: the U.S. Army studies using irradiation on rations.
- 1963: The United States approves irradiation of wheat and wheat flour and canned bacon.
- 1964: The United States approves irradiation of potatoes. No wheat or potatoes are sold, as producers are wary of scaring customers with mandatory labels reading "treated with gamma radiation."
- 1983: Food and Drug Administration approves irradiation of spices and seasonings. Less than 5 percent of spices are now irradiated.
- 1986: FDA approves irradiation of fresh fruits and vegetables. Law that such produce must be labeled. Dose approval: 1 kilGray, which is equal to 10 million chest X rays.
- October 1992: FDA approves irradiating poultry.

▲

"Food irradiation is supposed to preserve food. However, cancer-causing aflatoxin-producing molds, radiolytic by-products and 'free radicals' linked to cancer will be produced. A massive new health threat to U.S. citizens is set to begin."
—KARL GROSSMAN, *The Southampton Press*, September 5, 1991

▲

Be aware of the similarity between the logo for irradiated food and the logo for pure food:

The Radura   **The Logo for Purity**

The symbol for irradiated food (left), designed to let the consumer know that the food is irradiated, is very similar to the design of the symbol that is the logo of the Environmental Protection Agency, which is intended to denote purity.

▲

"Electromagnetic fields may interfere with the electrical chit-chat between cells in the body—and cooperate with carcinogens to disrupt normal regulation of cell growth and promote cancer development."
—*Science News*, Vol. 33, April 2, 1988

▲

ELECTROPOLLUTION

Another form of radiation is electromagnetic energy, which does not produce free radicals yet can be health damaging. All electrical devices produce some type of electric, magnetic, or electromagnetic fields. The frequency of these fields determines the biological effect on humans. Radiation, X rays, and ultraviolet radiation cause formation of free radicals. Low-frequency (ELF) fields do not do this, but there is abundant documentation that they do weaken health in a subtle but definite way.

EMR Upsets Body's Natural Magnetic Balance

Exposure to electromagnetic radiation (EMR) can upset the natural magnetic balance of the body and trigger mental and physical health problems. The function of cells is disordered when exposed to the stress of positive magnetic energy. The body requires a negative magnetic energy to maintain the alkaline body chemistry that is necessary to utilize oxygen. So when low-frequency fields switch the body chemistry to be more acidic than alkaline, pathogenic bacteria and viruses can gain a hold.

ELF	RADIO WAVES	MICROWAVES	INFRARED	VISIBLE LIGHT	ULTRA VIOLET	X-RAYS	GAMMA RAYS

LOW FREQUENCY
LONG WAVELENGTH

HIGH FREQUENCY
SHORT WAVELENGTH

▲

"Unless we change direction we are likely to
end up where we are headed."
—Chinese proverb

▲

Electromagnetic fields (EMF) and radiation (EMR) are all around us. They come from domestic appliances like TVs, stereos, VCRs, radios, toasters, fluorescent lights, electric blankets, microwave ovens, computers, and cellular phones, as well as from military installations, radar satellites, industrial machinery, radio and TV broadcast towers, electric light transformers, and high-current electric power lines. The potential for health damage is high. EMF and EMR have been linked to altered blood pressure, change in body chemistry resulting in less oxygen, a weakened immune system, changes in white and red blood cell counts, chronic fatigue, miscarriages, cancer, birth defects, depression, and learning disabilities. Over sixty studies link electromagnetic fields to cancer, leukemia, and tumors. In a research report in the *American Journal of Epidemiology* (Vol. 109, pp. 273–84, 1979) by Nancy Wertheimer, Ph.D., and Edward Leeper, Ph.D., it was observed that children living in homes near overhead electrical wires carrying high currents died of cancer at a rate *twice* that of those children living near low-current wiring. A Swedish study presented at the 1992 conference sponsored by the U.S. Department of Energy and the Electrical Power Research Institute found that children exposed to weak magnetic fields from power lines develop leukemia at almost *four* times the expected rate.

▲

"I believe I've found the missing link between
animal and civilized man. It is us."
—Konrad Lorenz

▲

The evidence makes protecting yourself from as much EMF and EMR exposure as you can a must. Check for transformers on wiring near your house. Test your home and work environment. Amplify your health through maintaining an alkaline body chemistry: ensure a diet emphasizing grains and vegetables and protective supplements (as outlined in Chapters 3 and 4). Reduce stress (which is acid forming) and ensure adequate oxygen.

WATER

Water, water everywhere, but is there a clean drop to drink? Water has been called the most important essential nutrient. Yet today water is full of chemicals and so is not something we can any longer use as an essential nutrient. These chemicals are free-radical-causing and health-depleting. Here are just some of the unwanted added ingredients drinking water may contain: aluminum salts, which may encourage development of Alzheimer's disease, 500 different chemicals from agriculture and industry, fluorides (which are immune-suppressing), chlorine (which can combine with other chemicals to form poisons), toxic levels of copper leached from copper pipes, lead from lead pipes or lead solder, plutonium, radioactive fallout, cadmium, and mercury. The potential for health damage is vast, including cancer, birth defects, genetic damage, weakened immunity, liver damage, and kidney damage.

▲

"Fluoride slows down and weakens those very cells which serve as the body's defense system and thus allows foreign agents such as bacteria, viruses, and chemicals as well as the body's own damaged or cancerous cells to wreak havoc throughout the body. Fluoride accelerates the aging process of the body."
—JOHN YIAMOUYIANNIS, *Fluoride: The Aging Factor*, Health Action Press, 1983

▲

The facts are grim: in 1982, 43 percent of American water violated federal health standards. The EPA has found unacceptable levels of lead in drinking water in 20 percent of cities, affecting in addition to the general population approximately 9 million children. Water is contaminated by 13,000 potentially toxic chemicals. Think of all this—and keep in mind that 75 percent of our body weight is water!

One major potential toxin in the water is fluoride, which is added to 60 percent of U.S. water for its cavity-preventing properties. But fluoride can also interfere with collagen formation, damage the immune system, destroy enzymes, cause mental lethargy, contribute to early aging, and weaken the thyroid gland. Fluoride is also found in toothpastes, fluoride treatments at the dentist, mouthwash, industrial pollution, and even bottled drinking water prepared specifically for babies.

Endangered Rivers of 1993

1. Rio Grande and Rio Conchos River System—Colorado, New Mexico, Texas, Mexico
2. Columbia and Snake River System, including the Yakima tributary—Northwest U.S., Canada
3. Everglades—Florida
4. Anacostia River—Washington, D.C., Maryland
5. Virgin River—Utah, Arizona, Nevada
6. Rogue and Illinois River System—Oregon
7. Penobscot River—Maine
8. Clavey River—California
9. Alsek and Tatshenshini River System—Alaska and British Columbia
10. Platte River—Nebraska

Water Filters

Since it is a given that most drinking water is not acceptable, what are the alternatives? Bottled water, or a water filter. The best bottled water is one that comes from a very deep and ancient source of water. Not surface water, or runoff from glaciers, both of which may contain toxins.

Types of Water Filters

Two main types are those connected under the sink to the cold water line or attached to the faucet above the sink.

Carbon Filtration

The simplest technique of filtration, which passes water through carbon, which captures contaminates.

Reverse Osmosis

This is a separation process that allows the water through a membrane while the contaminants go down the drain. It does not remove all bacteria or chemicals.

Combination of Filter and Reverse Osmosis

This combination does remove all undesirable contaminants. It is more expensive than the filter alone but it does a much better job. It also removes radioactive elements.

Distillation

This process of steaming off does remove most minerals and trace elements, but not all chemicals—and it leaves a depleted, denatured sort of water.

▲

"Despite growing interest in the fate of the
planet, nothing short of sharp changes will

rescue the Earth's ailing eco-systems from destruction.''
—The 1992 Annual Report of the WorldWatch Institute

▲

Now that you've read all about free radicals and our toxic world—and strategies for countering both—take a baseline assessment of your own health.

Questionnaire for an Assessment of Your Health Status

Answer the following questions. Then add up all the yes answers. Multiply by 2. 100 is a perfect score.

	YES	NO
Free Radicals (Part I)		
Do you know what free radicals are?	_____	_____
Do you know what causes free radicals?	_____	_____
Do you have no allergies?	_____	_____
Do you experience steady all-day energy?	_____	_____
Food (Chapter 3)		
Do you eat grains and vegetables and beans as your main meal four or more times a week?	_____	_____
Do you avoid sugar and foods with sugar?	_____	_____
Do you avoid meat, or limit to two times per week?	_____	_____
Do you avoid freshwater fish?	_____	_____
If you don't already grow your own vegetable garden, could you?	_____	_____
Do you eat mostly organic food?	_____	_____
Do you grow your own sprouts?	_____	_____
Do you easily maintain your ideal weight?	_____	_____

	YES	NO

Supplements (Chapter 4)

Do you take vitamin supplements
regularly?

Do you take antioxidants?

Do you take enzymes?

Do you take blue-green algae?

Do you take a detox supplement, such as
Kyolic?

Do you take free-radical-fighting enzymes
such as Cell Guard?

Do you take extra vitamin C when under
stress?

Do you drink herbal tea?

Do you have few, if any, brown spots?

Exercise (Chapter 5)

Do you exercise at least 45 minutes 3
times a week?

Do you do brisk walking outdoors 3 or
more times a week?

Do you practice yoga?

Do you do stretching exercises?

Do you lie on a slant board?

Do you play a sport?

Do you practice breathing exercises?

Do you do reflexology?

Mind Power (Chapter 6)

Do you know three ways to cope well with
stress?

Do you meditate daily?

Do you take breaks for deep breathing
during the day?

	YES	NO

Mind Power (Chapter 6) (*cont.*)

Do you have good concentration? _____ _____

Do you know two ways to generate health- _____ _____
building mental opiates?

Do you emphasize optimism? _____ _____

Do you take a break for laughter? _____ _____

Light (Chapter 7)

Do you spend one hour daily in daylight _____ _____
without glasses or contact lenses?

Do you avoid working under fluorescent _____ _____
light?

Do you avoid the midday sun? _____ _____

Do you avoid long sun exposure on the _____ _____
beach or water or in snow?

If you work in an office or at home do you _____ _____
make a point to take a full-spectrum
light break?

Pollution Avoidance (Chapter 8)

Do you drink filtered or bottled water? _____ _____

Do you avoid living less than thirty miles _____ _____
from a nuclear plant?

Do you avoid aluminum cookware? _____ _____

Do you avoid mercury fillings? _____ _____

Do you eat pesticide-free organic food? _____ _____

Do you avoid using pesticides in and _____ _____
around your home?

Do you eat low on the food chain (no dairy _____ _____
or meat)?

Do you take some actions to protect the _____ _____
earth?

YES   NO

Pollution Avoidance (Chapter 8)
  (*cont.*)
Are you aware of sources of   _____   _____
  electromagnetic pollution in your
  neighborhood?

Now that you know where you stand, make a plan for improvement.

Make a specific goal in each category (both long-range and short-term) and write it in the place provided.

Copy the chart on the next page for each month and tack it up someplace where you can write on it every day.

▲

"We discovered that the earth only *seems* flat, the sun only *seems* to circle the earth, matter only *seems* solid. Each of these discoveries is properly described as a paradigm shift."
—MARILYN FERGUSON, *Aquarian Conspiracy*, 1980

▲

Another paradigm shift has appeared: the understanding that there is a single cause of disease—that the free radical is the determinant of disease and health.

The traditional approach to health care has seen each disease as a separate entity, and treated symptoms out of their context. The new approach to health and well-being, as proposed in this book, sees all disease as related and addresses the whole person within their environment.

It is no longer necessary to look for a specific treatment for every ailment. Reducing the amount of pollutants produced and your exposure to existing ones, plus increasing the methods

Long-Range Health Goals:

Health Goal for This Month:

	Week 1	**Week 2**	**Week 3**	**Week 4**
Food				
Supplements				
Exercise				
Mind-Body				
Light				
Avoiding Pollution				

that counter excess free radicals discussed in the last six chapters are, together, the key to avoiding illness and creating health. The free radical is a contributing cause in every disease; and the free radical itself is a result of an overall imbalanced system. Treating the immediate cause will be effective if the prime cause is also attended to, in this case this would mean acknowledging the condition of our earth habitat and doing something about it immediately.

The following section, Part III, contains complete menus to give an idea of how to combine the beneficial foods into a meal. Part IV contains back-up information and leads to helpful resources.

Part III

COMPLETE MENUS FOR YOUTHFUL GOOD HEALTH

"Let food be your medicine, and medicine be your food."
—*Hippocrates*

MENUS AND RECIPES

These recipes are presented in groups forming menus for complete meals. The recipes contain the health-building foods (as described in Chapter 3), and the menus illustrate how to combine them and what the approximate proportions should be. The ratio between the types of foods is important; generally the grains and beans should comprise about 25 to 45 percent of the meal, with the balance being comprised of a variety of vegetables. It would be good to have about 20 percent of the meal be raw vegetables, sprouts, and greens so as to benefit from their enzymes and vital energy. The menus are presented by season to point out what foods are seasonal and the value of thinking of foods by their season.

It is recommended that the main meal be at midday. This gives time for digestion and is much better for overall health. If this is not possible, eat as many hours before sleeping as you can. Desserts may be eaten an hour or two after the meal if you like. The meals may seem generous. All the recipes are for four people and there is a variety of dishes, so if there are extras, someone will welcome them the next day. The recipes are designed to be simple to prepare with easily available ingredients, and not too many of them. A few of the foods might not be familiar to you. You'll find them in most health stores, or they can be purchased through the mail order food companies listed in Part IV.

Instructions for making the sprouts, which are included in almost every meal, follow the recipes. Give them a try—they have great value, being clean, home-grown, and organic, and fresh and vital. A plus is they are inexpensive. Also following the recipes are a few supporting suggestions, a tea and a few condiments that can be healthfully and tastefully sprinkled on a rice or vegetable dish to enhance its sparkle.

Of course, keep in mind that organic foods are better for you. So try to use as many organic foods as you can. Many cities have organic markets, or an organic section in the supermarket. You can send for organic foods by mail (see Part IV for resources). And, creating your own garden, even if only for a few items, is a wonderful idea. The food in these recipes is from the lower end of the food chain. Foods that are high on the food chain, such as meat and dairy products, contain a greater concentration of pesticides and toxins, so they are best avoided. A varied and balanced meal of grains, beans, and vegetables with occasional fruit is delicious, nutrifying, and also low on the food chain.

You will notice there is no sugar used, as this is a nonnutrifying and depleting food. Some good oils are used and oils are necessary for health (contrary to the popular rush to avoid all oils). Moderation is the key. A pinch of salt is also necessary for health, and the salt in these recipes is balanced by its partner, potassium, which is found in many vegetables. Be sure to use good, clean filtered water or spring water. Tap water has too many chemicals in it.

Completely avoid all aluminum cooking utensils and be sure you have stainless steel pans and a good heavy iron skillet.

These recipes will provide you with some delicious meals. And they will also introduce you to a selection of key foods and their best ratio in a meal. I wish you good appetite and optimum health!

A Winter Menu (1)

Try this version of "mashed potatoes" made with millet and cauliflower. Along with the sauté of spinach and carrot-sprout salad you have a fine meal. And, it's easy to make in a half hour. Make the strawberry pudding ahead so it will have time to chill.

Winter Soup with Onion, Tofu, and Miso

Delicious Millet "Mashed Potatoes"

Sauté of Spinach and Turnips

Refurbishing Sprouts and Carrot Salad

Strawberry Pudding

✽ *Winter Soup with Onion, Tofu, and Miso*

1 t. sesame oil
1½ cups onion, finely chopped
5 cups water, filtered or spring
4-inch piece of wakame, rinsed and soaked 5 minutes and
   sliced
2 t. miso
1 cup tofu, finely cubed
3–4 T. scallions, finely chopped

Sauté onions in heavy saucepan until tender. Add water and wakame. Bring to a boil. Stir in tofu, reduce heat, and simmer 2 minutes. Blend a few tablespoons of the broth with the miso in a cup and return to the pot. Serve garnished with scallions.

Serves: 4
Time: 10 minutes

❧ *Delicious Millet "Mashed Potatoes"*

1 cup millet
2½ cups water, filtered or spring
½ medium-size cauliflower, sliced into thin pieces
½ t. sea salt
3 cloves garlic, cut in pieces
1 T. olive oil
3 T. fresh lemon juice
2 T. water
pinch sea salt
pinch freshly ground pepper
1 T. parsley, finely chopped

Rinse the millet and drain. Slice the cauliflower into thin pieces so it will cook with the millet. Put the water, millet, cauliflower, and garlic into a heavy saucepan and cook for 7 minutes on medium heat. Take pan off the heat, cover, and let sit for 20 minutes to steam. Mash well with a potato masher. Blend the olive oil, lemon juice, water, salt and pepper and add to the mashed millet and combine well. Serve sprinkled with finely chopped parsley.

Serves: 4
Time: 30 minutes

❧ Sauté of Spinach and Turnip

1 large bunch spinach, washed and cleaned, stems removed
2 turnips, peeled and cut into matchstick slices
2 T. canola oil
3 T. lemon juice
pinch sea salt
pinch freshly ground pepper

In a large skillet, heat the oil. Add the sliced turnips and cook until browned. Add the spinach and cook until it is wilted. Add the lemon juice and salt and pepper. Transfer to a warmed serving bowl.

Serves: 4
Time: 10 minutes

🐚 *Refurbishing Sprouts and Carrot Salad*

2 cups sprouts, whatever kind you have on hand
2 cups grated carrots
¼ cup parsley, finely chopped
3 T. lemon juice
2 T. olive oil
1 T. Braggs (optional) Liquid Aminos
pinch cayenne

Put salad ingredients in serving bowl. Blend dressing ingredients in small bowl. Whisk to blend. Toss dressing and salad and let sit 20 minutes before serving.

Serves: 4
Time: 25 minutes

🐚 *Strawberry Pudding*

1½ cups frozen organic strawberries
1½ cups tofu
2 T. maple syrup
2 t. vanilla extract

Put all ingredients into a blender and puree. Put into medium-size bowl, cover, and refrigerate for about an hour before serving.

Serves: 4
Time: 1 hour

A Winter Menu (2)

Polenta, greens with garlic, spicy black beans,
and sprout salad make a hearty meal.

Warming Vegetable Health-Building Soup

Polenta

Spicy Black Beans

Kale and Collards with Garlic

Home-Grown Winter Sprout Salad

Lovely Lemon Pudding

🍂 *Warming Vegetable Health-Building Soup*

1½ T. olive oil
½ cup onions, finely chopped
1 clove garlic, chopped
1 cup carrots, sliced into rounds
4 cups water, filtered or spring
1 cup zucchini, cut in half lengthwise and then into half
  rounds
1 cup cabbage, thinly sliced
½ t. dried thyme
½ t. oregano
½ t. sea salt
2-inch strip of kombu
3 t. miso
½ cup parsley, minced

Sauté the oil, onions, and garlic in a heavy soup pot. Add the water, carrots, zucchini, cabbage, kombu, and spices. Simmer 5 to 7 minutes or until cabbage softens. Add parsley, stir to blend, and serve.

Serves: 4
Time: 15–20 minutes

🍂 *Polenta*

3 cups water, filtered or spring
1 T. corn or canola oil
½ t. sea salt
1 cup yellow cornmeal
1 cup cold water, filtered or spring

Boil 3 cups of water in heavy 2-quart saucepan. Add the oil and salt. Combine cornmeal and cup of water in medium-size bowl. Add the cornmeal mixture to the boiling water while stirring. Whisk constantly. When mixture returns to boil, turn down the heat and cook uncovered for about 20–25 minutes. Stir frequently. Mixture will be the consistency of heavy mashed potatoes.

Lightly oil a $9 \times 9 \times 2$ pan. Pour the cornmeal mixture into the pan and let it set. After half an hour or more it will be firm enough to cut.

Cut down the middle, and then cut each half into thirds. Serve one of the six portions to each, reserving the two seconds for the next day's lunch. The leftover polenta can be lightly brushed with oil and put under the broiler until browned, about 4 minutes on each side. Good with a quick steamed vegetable and miso broth.

Serves: 4
Time: 1 hour

🍂 *Spicy Black Beans*

2 cups black beans, sorted and well rinsed
6 cups water, filtered or spring
3–6 cloves garlic, crushed
1 medium onion, diced
2 t. chili powder or less to taste
½ cup cooking liquid reserved
1 T. olive oil
1 red onion, finely chopped

Soak beans in water to cover overnight or 8 hours. Rinse a reserve ½ cup of cooking liquid. Cook beans in water to cover for 1 hour or until tender. In a large skillet sauté the garlic and onion about 5 minutes in the olive oil. Add the chili powder, stir to mix. Add the cooked beans, ½ cup water, and cook uncovered for about 5 minutes until sauce thickens. Serve topped with diced red onion.

Serves: 4
Time: 8 hours baking; 1 hour cooking

🐝 *Kale and Collards with Garlic*

4 cups fresh kale, torn into bite-size pieces
3 cups collards, torn into bite-size pieces
2 T. olive oil
4 cloves garlic
1 t. sea salt
pinch cayenne
2 t. cumin
3 t. lemon juice
pinch freshly ground pepper
3 T. parsley or cilantro, finely chopped
½ t. gomasio (optional recipe in back of this section)

Wash greens well. Steam the greens in a large steamer. (Cook collards first; they take longer than kale.) Five minutes should make the greens crunchy yet tender. Put the greens in a large colander and drain well. In a heavy skillet, put the oil, garlic, cayenne, cumin and stir to cook lightly for 2 minutes. Add the greens and toss and blend with the oil mixture to cover. Transfer to a large serving bowl and sprinkle with lemon juice. Top with some gomasio, if you like.

Serves: 4
Time: 10 minutes

❧ *Home-Grown Winter Sprout Salad*

2 cups any sprouts you have on hand (alfalfa, lentil,
   sunflower, or other)
1 cucumber, diced
2–3 scallions, chopped
3 T. lemon juice
2 T. tahini
1 t. Braggs Aminos
1 clove garlic, minced with ½ t. salt
pinch cayenne
pinch sea salt

    Put the salad ingredients in a serving bowl. In a small
bowl mix the lemon juice, tahini, Braggs, and garlic minced
with the salt. Add pinch of cayenne. Whisk together well. Pour
dressing over salad and toss to blend flavors.

Serves: 4
Time: 5 minutes

❧ *Lovely Lemon Pudding*

3 cups apple juice
3 T. agar flakes
¼ cup maple syrup
¼ t. turmeric (for coloring)
pinch sea salt
3 T. kuzu
½ cup water
1 t. vanilla extract
2 t. lemon zest (grated lemon rind)
½ cup fresh lemon juice
1 cup berries (optional)

In a heavy saucepan, mix the apple juice, agar, maple syrup, turmeric, and salt. Cook over medium heat for 5–10 minutes until the agar is completely dissolved. Stir occasionally. In a small bowl, mix the kuzu and water and vanilla. Add the kuzu mixture to the cooking pot and cook until slightly thickened, approximately 5 minutes. Remove from heat and add lemon juice and lemon zest. Pour into dessert cups and let set for about an hour.

You can top with any fresh berries. Or it is equally good on its own.

Serves: 4
Time: 15 minutes
   1 hour to set

A Spring Menu (1)

A charming, healthful meal in 25 minutes.

Spring Soup with Miso and Spinach

Parsleyed Millet

Tasty Carrots

Stir-fried Tofu with Broccoli

Spring Dandelion and Sprout Salad

Strawberry Sherbet

❧ Spring Soup with Miso and Spinach

5 cups water, filtered or spring
1 5-inch strip of kombu
1 bunch spinach, washed well and shredded
1 cup tofu, finely diced
2 t. miso (½ t. per serving)
2 T. lemon juice

Boil water with kombu for 5 minutes. Remove kombu and save for the next soup. Add washed spinach and simmer covered for 2 minutes. Add the tofu and simmer for 2 minutes. Blend the miso with a few tablespoons of the hot broth in a small cup and return to the pot. Stir. Add the lemon juice and serve.

Serves: 4
Time: 10 minutes

੨ঌ *Parsleyed Millet*

1 cup millet
2 cups water, filtered or spring
pinch sea salt
¼ cup parsley, finely minced
gomasio (optional—recipe at end of this section)

Rinse the millet well. Add the millet to the water in a heavy saucepan and cook 5 minutes uncovered. Remove from the heat; add the minced parsley. Cover and let sit for 20 minutes. Toss with a fork to blend and serve. Sprinkle with gomasio (optional).

Serve: 4
Time: 25 minutes

≈ *Tasty Carrots*

4 carrots, rinsed, scrubbed, and cut into ⅛-inch rounds
  slightly on the diagonal
½ cup orange juice (or ¼ cup lemon juice and ¼ cup water)
1 T. maple syrup
dash cayenne
pinch sea salt
½ t. fresh grated ginger (optional)

Put the carrots in a heavy saucepan. Mix the juice and the maple syrup in a cup and add to the carrots. Cook over low heat for about 5–7 minutes or until crisp-tender. Add the grated ginger, if you like the flavor, toward the end of cooking.

Serves: 4
Time: 10 minutes

≈ *Stir-fried Tofu with Broccoli*

1 cup tofu, crumbled
3 cups broccoli, cut into small pieces
1–2 t. sesame oil
1 large onion, finely chopped
pinch sea salt
1 t. gomasio (optional)

Add oil to a heavy skillet. Sauté the onions for about 5 minutes. Add the tofu and sauté for 1 minute. Add the broccoli to the mixture and cover the pan and cook for 3 minutes. Add salt.

Serves: 4
Time: 15 minutes

❧ Spring Dandelion and Sprout Salad

2 cups dandelions, well rinsed and chopped
2 cups sprouts, any kind you have on hand
¼ cup sunflower seeds (optional)
3 T. sesame oil
1½ T. umeboshi vinegar
1 t. lemon juice
½ t. Dijon mustard
pinch sea salt
pinch freshly ground pepper

Wash the dandelion well and cut into pieces. Put into bowl and refrigerate. Put the sprouts into a bowl and cover with the sauce and mix. Refrigerate 20 minutes or more to blend the flavors. When ready to serve, mix the sprouts with the dandelion in a serving bowl. Sprinkle with lemon juice.

Optional addition:
½ cup sunflower seeds

Place sunflower seeds in a heavy skillet and toast for 4–5 minutes, stirring and shaking the pan. Remove and put on a plate and sprinkle with Braggs Aminos. Let cool and add to salad just before serving.

Serves: 4
Time: 10 minutes
    Refrigerate sprouts 20 minutes

❧ *Strawberry Sherbet*

3 cups frozen organic strawberries, or fresh if available
1 banana, frozen, cut into chunks
3–4 T. vanilla yogurt

Put ingredients into a blender and blend until smooth. Put into dessert dishes and serve immediately. To freeze the banana, cut into chunks and place in plastic bag. Refrigerate 4–8 hours.

Serves: 4
Time: 5 minutes
    4 hours for freezing

A Spring Menu (2)

This vegetable stir-fry could be called the anti-oxidant special, filled as it is with beneficial broccoli, cauliflower, and carrots. The sprout salad supplies enzymes. The cornbread supplies some delicious crunchiness. A lovely meal ready in less than an hour. Prepare the apricot dessert ahead so it will have time to cool.

Heartening Broth

Cornbread

Delicious Brown Rice and Mixed-Vegetable Stir-fry

Sprout Salad

Poached Apricots

This broth contains sodium, referred to as the "youth element." Save the leftovers for a vitalizing snack the following day.

❧ Heartening Broth

1 cup carrots, chopped
2 cups carrot tops, chopped
3 cups celery stalks, chopped
1 onion, diced
3-inch piece of kombu
2 quarts water, filtered or spring
2 t. miso

Place all ingredients into a large heavy saucepan. Cover and cook for 20 minutes on medium heat. Strain. Add ½ teaspoon of miso per serving. Blend the miso with 2 tablespoons of the broth and then add to the pot after the soup has been strained.

Serves: 4
Time: 30 minutes

❧ Corn Bread

¾ cup cornmeal
¼ cup whole wheat pastry flour
¼ cup unbleached white flour
1 T. baking powder
pinch sea salt
5 T. canola or safflower oil
1 egg, beaten
⅓ cup maple syrup
1 cup soymilk or rice milk
2 t. oil

Preheat oven to 375°. Mix corn meal, the flour, and baking powder in a medium-size bowl. In a separate bowl mix the oil, egg, maple syrup, and soymilk. Add wet ingredients to dry ingredients, and mix only until blended. Lightly cover either an 8-inch iron skillet or an 8 × 8 pan with oil. Spoon in the batter. Bake about 35 minutes or until lightly browned. Is done when a toothpick inserted into the center emerges clean. Cut into squares and serve warm.

Serves: 8 (1 piece each)
Time: 45 minutes

🫖 *Delicious Brown Rice and Mixed-Vegetable Stir-fry*

1½ T. sesame oil
½ lb. tofu, cut into 1-inch cubes
2 T. Braggs Aminos
½ cup onion, diced
2 T. scallions, chopped
1 cup broccoli, cut into flowercttcs
1 cup cauliflower, sliced rather thinly
1 cup carrots, cut into ⅛-inch rounds
1½ cups cooked brown rice
3 cups water, filtered or spring
¼ cup parsley, finely chopped
sesame wakame condiment (recipe at end of this section)

Cook the brown rice in a heavy saucepan for about 45 minutes. Sprinkle the Braggs Aminos liquid over the cubed tofu and let stand 10 minutes. Heat oil in a heavy skillet or wok. Stir-fry the tofu for 4 minutes and remove from the pan. Boil large pot of water and blanch the vegetables for 1 minute in the boiling water. Strain the vegetables in a colander. Add the onions and scallions to the skillet. Cook 2 minutes. Add the blanched vegetables and cook 5 minutes or so until tender crisp. Add the cooked rice and cover and cook together 1 minute. Add the cooked tofu and stir-fry briefly. Add the chopped parsley. Place into a warmed serving dish and sprinkle with sesame wakame.

Serves: 4
Time: 50 minutes

❧ *Sprout Salad*

2 cups mixed sprouts, alfalfa, sunflower greens, lentils, or
  what you have on hand
1 cup red cabbage, finely chopped
1 cup celery, chopped
1 cup watercress or spinach, chopped
3 T. olive oil
2 T. lemon juice
dash cayenne
pinch sea salt
½ t. Dijon mustard

    Mix the salad ingredients in a serving bowl. In a small bowl mix the oil, lemon juice, cayenne, salt, and mustard. Add to the salad and mix well. Let stand to blend a few minutes before serving.

Serves: 4
Time: 10 minutes

❧ *Poached Apricots*

1 lb ripe yet firm apricots
3 cups water, filtered or spring
4 t. good honey
2 T. lemon juice
2 strips of lemon peel about 2 inches long
½ t. vanilla extract
2 very thin slices of fresh ginger or ½ t. powdered ginger

Rinse the apricots. Cut them in half and remove the pits. In a heavy saucepan, combine the water, honey, lemon juice and strips, ginger, and vanilla, and bring to a light simmer. Add the apricots and simmer on low heat for 5 minutes or until apricots are tender. Remove the apricots and set aside. Continue to simmer the syrup for about 20 minutes until it is reduced to about 1 cup. Pour the syrup over the apricots and refrigerate covered. Let come to room temperature before serving.

Serves: 4
Time: 25 minutes
    1 hour to cool

A Summer Menu (1)

This is a quick meal to prepare—30 minutes.
The colors—yellow, orange, green, red, and
blue—almost fill out the spectrum. And the
nutrients are equally satisfying.

Vital Broth

Tasty Millet Salad with Cashews and Currants

Watercress with Creamy Tofu Salad Dressing

Summer Carrot Salad with Bean Sprouts

Strawberry-Blueberry Compote

❧ *Vital Broth*

2 cups vegetable parings, or a mix of celery, carrot, onion,
   and any leftover greens
1 3-inch strip of kombu
6 cups water, filtered or spring
2 t. miso

    Boil the above covered for 20 minutes. Drain the broth.
Place a few sprigs of watercress and a few tiny cubes of the
tofu into the bottom of 4 soup cups and pour the hot broth
over. Let cool a bit before serving.

Serves: 6
Time: 30 minutes

❧ *Tasty Millet Salad with Cashews and Currants*

1½ cups millet
3 cups water, filtered or spring
⅓ cup currants (or raisins)
½ cup cashews, chopped in bits
1 T. sesame oil
3 T. lemon juice
1 T. lemon zest (grated lemon peel)
½ t. sea salt
2 t. mild curry powder
½ t. cumin
1 T. parsley
few sprigs watercress

Rinse the millet in a strainer and add to the water. Bring to a boil uncovered and cook for 5 minutes. Remove from heat, cover, and let sit for 20 minutes. In heavy frying pan, put the oil and the curry powder, cumin, and cayenne, stir to blend. Add the cashews and blend. Add the cooked millet and blend. Add the currants and sprinkle on the lemon zest and the lemon juice. Remove the mixture to a serving dish and let it cool to room temperature. Top with the parsley and serve.

Serves: 4
Time: 30 minutes

❧ Watercress with Creamy Tofu Salad Dressing

2 large bunches of watercress, finely chopped, about 3 cups
½ cup celery, finely diced
1 small red onion, thinly sliced
½ cup dulse, rinsed, soaked, and chopped in small pieces

Wash the watercress well and chop rather finely. Dice the celery. Slice the red onion into thin rings and then halve them. Place everything in a mixing bowl.

Dressing:
½ cup tofu
2 t. umeboshi plum vinegar
3 t. dill, chopped finely
2 t. lemon juice

Blend the tofu, umeboshi vinegar, dill, and lemon juice in a blender or mash well by hand to blend. Pour over the watercress salad and toss to mix well.

Serves: 4
Time: 10 minutes

৵ *Summer Carrot Salad with Bean Sprouts*

1 lb carrots (about 2 cups)
1 cup bean sprouts

Dressing:
3 T. lemon juice
1–2 T. olive oil
¼ t. paprika
3 t. fresh dill (or 1 t. dried)

Wash the carrots well. Lightly peel or brush with a strong vegetable brush. Grate the carrots with a carrot grater, or put through a food processor. Put the carrots and sprouts into a medium-size serving bowl. In a small bowl mix the salad dressing ingredients. Pour them over the salad and toss.

Serves: 4
Time: 10 minutes

🍃 *Strawberry-Blueberry Compote*

1 pint strawberries
1 pint blueberries
2–3 T. lemon or lime juice
1 T. maple syrup (honey will also do)
2 T. hazelnuts, chopped

Wash the berries well. Slice the strawberries, and take the stem off the blueberries. Put berries in a medium-size bowl. Combine the lemon juice and the syrup in a small bowl. Pour over and blend with the berries. Sprinkle hazelnuts on top.

Serves: 4
Time: 10 minutes

A Summer Menu (2)

This cool summer menu starts with a light broth. The rice salad is complemented by two salad dishes, stringbeans, and mixed arugula with sprouts. Peaches are featured in the ice-cream-like fruit puree for dessert.

Refreshing Dulse Broth

Rice Salad with Chickpeas

Sparkling Arugula, Red Onion, and Corn Salad with Sprouts

Stringbeans with Parsley Dressing

Peach Banana Puree

ঽ Refreshing Dulse Broth

4 cups water, filtered or spring
1 medium-size onion, chopped
1 cup dulse, chopped
1 fresh raw carrot, grated
2 t. miso (or 1¼ t. Braggs Aminos)

Boil the water and add the chopped onions and cook for 2 minutes. Add the dulse and the grated carrot. Cover and turn off the heat and let sit a few minutes to soften the carrot and dulse. Add the miso blended with some broth or Braggs Aminos liquid and stir to blend. Let come to almost room temperature and serve in small soup cups.

Serves: 4
Time: 10 minutes

❧ *Rice Salad with Chickpeas*

1½ cups long-grain brown rice
3 cups water, filtered or spring
1 1-inch piece of kombu, broken in bits
2 t. dried oregano, finely crumbled
¾ cup cooked chickpeas
3 T. chopped chives or finely chopped scallions
¼ cup parsley, finely chopped

Dressing:
2 T. freshly squeezed lemon juice
¼ cup olive oil
½ t. Tabasco, or to taste
½ t. sea salt
1½ t. Dijon mustard

Boil 3 cups water. Add the bits of kombu and rice. Bring to a boil, reduce heat, cover, and simmer on low heat for about 45 minutes. Mix the ingredients for the dressing together. Whisk to blend well and refrigerate. When rice is cooked, pour in a large bowl and let cool a bit. (It can be made ahead, but be sure to bring to room temperature before serving.) Add the dressing to the rice. Add the chickpeas and chives and parsley and mix all together.

Serves: 4
Time: 1 hour

🐦 Sparkling Arugula, Red Onion, and Corn Salad with Sprouts

2 cups arugula, well washed and chopped into bite-size
  pieces
2 cups cooked corn (about 3 ears)
1 large red onion, thinly sliced
1 cup sprouts, whatever you have on hand

Dressing:
2 T. tahini
2 t. light miso
¼ cup water, filtered or spring
¼ cup fresh lemon juice
pinch cayenne
pinch sea salt
pinch freshly ground pepper
2 T. fresh dill from the garden or 2 t. dried dill

Mix the miso in with the water, then add the tahini and mix well. Add the lemon juice and the cayenne, salt, pepper, and fresh dill. Blend all together. Wash the arugula well. Boil a big pot of water and cook the 3 ears of fresh corn for 3–4 minutes until just done. Remove from water and cool. With a sharp knife, remove the corn kernels from the ear. Slice the red onion very thin. Put the arugula in a nice serving bowl; add the corn and the red onion. Pour the dressing over and toss to mix well.

Serves: 4
Time: 10 minutes

❧ Stringbeans with Parsley Dressing

4 cups stringbeans, or broad Italian beans, trimmed and cut
on diagonal

Dressing:
¼ cup parsley, finely minced
1 T. olive oil
2 T. fresh lemon juice
pinch sea salt
pinch freshly ground pepper
1 lemon, cut into 4 pieces

Steam the stringbeans for about 5 minutes until tender yet
still crunchy. Rinse with cool water and put in mixing bowl.
Mix the lemon juice, oil, and parsley together. Pour over the
string beans and toss together. Serve with extra lemon wedges.

Serves: 4
Time: 10 minutes

❧ *Peach Banana Puree*

4 ripe peaches
2 ripe bananas
¼ cup yogurt
1 t. vanilla extract
1 T. maple syrup (optional)
1 t. freshly grated nutmeg (optional)

Peal the peaches and cut into chunks. Cut the bananas into chunks. Freeze in a plastic bag 4–8 hours. Put peaches and bananas in blender or food processor and process until almost smooth. Serve in dessert dishes. Grate some nutmeg on top if you like.

Serves: 4
Time: 10 minutes preparation
4–8 hours in freezer

A Fall Menu (1)

This hearty autumn meal will be ready in less than an hour and features millet formed in croquettes with two fall vegetables—a green and a yellow—and a traditional apple dessert.

Delicious Split Pea Soup

Millet Croquettes with Dipping Sauce

Mashed Yellow Acorn Squash

Leafy Greens Steamed

Grandma's Apple Crumble

🏺 *Delicious Split Pea Soup*

Such a simple and tasty soup! With the addition of celery and carrots the potassium supplies are increased and the soup is nicely thickened. If you want to double the recipe, you will have some for the next day's lunch.

1 cup split peas
6 cups water, filtered or spring
1 4-inch piece of wakame
1 onion, diced
3 cloves garlic
1 cup celery, diced
1 cup carrot, diced
pinch sea salt
3 scallions, chopped

Add all the ingredients to a large heavy pot. Bring to a boil, cover, and simmer 30 minutes. Mash cooked peas and vegetables with a heavy fork against the side of the pot, or put half the mixture into a blender and then replace in pot. Sprinkle with chopped scallions.

Serves: 4
Time: 30 minutes

❧ *Millet Croquettes with Dipping Sauce*

This millet patty can compete with and outdo a hamburger. The herbs give the naturally bland millet oomph and the sauté in oil and onion gives a crunchy exterior. Dip in some sauce and you have a taste treat.

1 cup millet
2 cups water, filtered or spring
1 small onion
2 T. sesame or safflower oil
3 T. parsley, minced
2 scallions, thinly sliced
½ t. marjoram
½ t. basil
½ t. sage
(or in place of the above 3, 1½ t. Italian mixed herbs)

Cook millet in water for 5 minutes. Take off the heat, cover, and let sit for 20 minutes. Blend millet with scallion and herbs in mixing bowl. Wet your hands so mixture won't stick, and shape into patties. Chop onion finely and sauté in oil in a heavy skillet until lightly browned. Sauté patties in skillet until browned on both sides.

Dipping Sauce:
1 T. soy sauce
4 T. rice vinegar
2 T. sake or white wine

Combine ingredients and mix together. Place in several small dishes for dipping or spoon over the croquettes.

Serves: 4
Time: 35 minutes

ᘒ Mashed Yellow Acorn Squash

Seasonal squash served up like mashed potatoes. The color is sparkling and the squash is loaded with wonderful vitamin A.

3 medium/large acorn squash
3 t. tamari
pinch sea salt

Cut the squash in half and deseed. Place cut side down on cookie sheet in a preheated oven at 350° for 45–50 minutes. Scoop squash out of the shells. Add tamari, a pinch of salt, and blend with potato masher or heavy fork until mashed.

Serves: 4
Time: 50 minutes

ᘒ Leafy Greens Steamed

No one will have to say "eat your greens." Simply steamed and sprinkled with lemon, leafy greens couldn't be better.

6–8 cups kale or other leafy greens
juice of 1 fresh lemon

Wash greens well. Remove tough stems. Chop into bite-size pieces. Steam in large double boiler for about 5 minutes. Turn into pot or serving bowl and sprinkle with lemon juice.

Serves: 4
Time: 10 minutes

❧ *Grandma's Apple Crumble*

It always seemed that a good apple dessert needed sugar. This one is sweetened just enough with maple syrup and tarted just enough with lemon. This under a crunchy oat topping makes a satisfying finish to a deliciously distinctive fall meal.

6 medium apples
2 T. lemon juice
1 T. lemon rind
½ t. cinnamon
2 T. safflower oil
½ cup maple syrup
⅓ cup whole wheat or oat flour
pinch sea salt
⅔ cup rolled oats
1 t. vanilla extract

Peel and slice the apples. Grease a shallow baking dish. Place the apples in the dish with lemon juice, rind, and cinnamon. Mix oil, salt, flour, maple syrup, and oats together and sprinkle over apples. Bake in oven at 325° for about 40 minutes. Let cool a bit before serving.

Serves: 4
Time: 50 minutes

A Fall Menu (2)

This meal contains a wonderful variety of vegetables from the spinach in the soup to the three-vegetable dish to the sprout salad. This abundance is well balanced by the lentils and the crunchy rice patties. All rounded off with a grape-colored dessert.

If you prepare the rice ahead and the kanten dessert ahead, preparation time for dinner will only be 50 minutes.

Popeye and Olive Oyl Spinach Soup

Vegetable Delight: Red Cabbage, Scallions, and Cauliflower

Rice Patties

Sunny Salad

Grape Kanten

Oatmeal Pecan Cookies

❧ *Popeye and Olive Oyl Spinach Soup*

1 onion, chopped
2 T. olive oil
2 cups lentils
½ t. thyme
5 cups water, filtered or spring
½ t. basil
pinch cayenne
pinch chili powder
1 big bunch spinach, well washed and chopped
2 cloves garlic, chopped
¼ cup fresh lemon juice
¼ cup fresh basil leaves, chopped (if available)

Sauté the onion in the oil in a heavy soup pot. Add water and bring to a boil. Add lentils and return to boil. Add spices. Cover and cook about 40 minutes or until lentils are tender. Add chopped spinach, garlic, and lemon juice. Cover, simmer 1 minute.

Serves: 4
Time: 50 minutes

❧ Vegetable Delight: Red Cabbage, Scallions, and Cauliflower

1 cup red cabbage, finely chopped
1 cup scallions, sliced on the diagonal
1 cup cauliflower, finely sliced
½ cup cashew bits
¼ cup cilantro, finely chopped
¼ cup raisins
cooking broth or water, filtered or spring
4 t. Braggs Liquid Aminos (or 2 t. miso)
1 T. olive oil

Put water, Braggs Aminos, and oil in a heavy skillet and heat through. Add the vegetables and cook over medium heat, stirring to mix. Cook about 5–7 minutes. If using miso, blend water with it and add after mixture is cooked.

Serves: 4–5
Time: 25 minutes

🍂 Rice Patties

2 T. olive oil
1 cup short-grain brown rice
2 cups water, filtered or spring
1 medium-large onion, finely chopped
2 T. whole wheat flour
1 egg, beaten to blend
¼ cup parsley, finely chopped
1½ T. olive oil
¼ cup dulse, soaked 5 minutes and diced
pinch sea salt
pinch freshly ground black pepper
pinch cayenne

Cook the rice in the water in a heavy saucepan for 45 minutes or till done. Place the oil in a small saucepan, add the onion, and cook for about 5 minutes. Put the cooked rice and flour in a medium-size bowl and stir to coat the rice with the flour. Add the egg, salt, pepper, cayenne, parsley, and cooked onion and mix together. Form 8 patties about 3 inches across. Put them on a cookie sheet and refrigerate for about one hour so that they set. Put the olive oil in a heavy skillet over moderate heat. Put the patties in the skillet and cook until golden, about 2 minutes on each side.

Serves: 4
Time:*

---

*The rice can be cooked ahead and formed into patties. If so, cooking time is about 16 minutes if you do 2 batches of 4 patties in your skillet.

🍂 *Sunny Salad*

1 cup sunflower sprouts (or whatever is on hand)
1 cup watercress, well washed and finely chopped
1 T. sesame oil
3 T. lemon juice
1 t. umeboshi plum paste

Put the sprouts and watercress in serving bowl. In a small bowl, mix the lemon juice and umeboshi paste together. Drizzle in the oil and blend. Pour over the salad and let sit to blend flavors for 15 minutes.

Serves: 4
Time: 20 minutes

❧ Grape Kanten

2 cups apple juice
2 cups grape juice
3 T. agar flakes
¼ cup water, filtered or spring
3 T. kuzu

In a heavy saucepan, mix the apple juice, grape juice, and agar. Cook over medium heat 5–10 minutes until agar is completely dissolved. Stir occasionally. In a small bowl mix the water and kuzu. Add the kuzu mixture to the pot and stir until thickened, about 5 minutes. Remove from heat. Pour into dessert cups and allow about an hour to settle before serving.

Serves: 4
Time: 10 minutes
*   1 hour to set*

❧ *Oatmeal Pecan Cookies*

1¼ cup pastry flour
1¼ cup rolled oats
1 cup pecans, chopped into bits
pinch sea salt
½ cup corn oil
½ cup rice syrup
2 t. vanilla extract
1 t. canola oil

Combine the flour, oats, and pecans in a medium-size bowl. Mix the syrup and oil and vanilla together. Add the syrup mixture to the flour mixture and blend but do not mix more than just enough to blend. Lightly oil with canola or corn oil on a cookie sheet. Heat oven to 350°. Put rounded teaspoons of cookie dough onto cookie sheet. If you put them into the shape you want they will hold to it. At the rate of 1 t. of batter per cookie, it will make approximately 30 cookies. Bake for 12 minutes. Keep a watch on them, as every oven varies.

Serve: 15
Time: 25 minutes

MORE RECIPES

Following are some suggestions: a tea, two condiments, and directions for making your own sprouts.

❧ *Kombu Tea*

1 3-inch strip of kombu
1 quart water, filtered or spring

Put the kombu in a heavy pot with the water and boil for 10 minutes. This makes a strengthening tea.

Serves: 4
Time: 10 minutes

❧ *Gomasio—Sea Salt with Sesame Seeds*

This is wonderful sprinkled on rice or vegetables. Keep a batch on the shelf in a tightly closed glass jar to preserve its sparkling favor.

1 cup black sesame seeds
1½–2 T. sea salt

Toast the salt in a heavy iron frying pan over a low heat. Stir carefully with a wooden spoon 1–2 minutes. Pour into a heavy dish and crush with back of spoon. Use a suribachi if you have one. Wash and drain the sesame seeds. Wipe out the frying pan and use it to roast the seeds over a low flame. Stir occasionally with a wooden spoon. The seeds will darken and give off a nutty fragrance. When a seed is easy to crush between your fingers, then it is done. Pour the seeds into the bowl with the salt. Grind and mash the two together. Continue until about half the seeds are crushed. Let mixture cool and pour into a glass jar or container with tight-fitting lid.

🐤 *Sesame and Wakame*

4–5 10-inch strips of wakame
½ cup whole sesame seeds

Put unwashed dry wakame on a baking sheet in the oven at 350° and bake for 15 minutes. Wash and drain the sesame seeds. Put them in a heavy frying pan over a low heat and stir with a wooden spoon. When seeds give off a nutty fragrance and begin to pop, test by squeezing one between your fingers to see if it will crush easily. If it does, it is ready. Pour into a bowl. Remove wakame from the oven and crumble it into small pieces in a heavy mixing bowl. Grind to a powder. (If you have a mortar or pestle, use it. Otherwise a clay or glass mixing bowl and a wooden spoon will do.) Add the seeds and grind together until half the seeds are crushed. Let cool and pour mixture into a glass jar with a tight lid. Sprinkle on grains or salads or vegetables.

SPROUTS

Sprouts are the first growth of a plant from seeds, which go from a dormant state to a live state by the addition of water. Sprouts are a special food for the free-radical-fighting food plan because they contain abundant nutrients, enzymes, and chlorophyll while being a noncontaminated food due to the fact they are grown from organic seeds, with filtered or spring water with no chemicals whatsoever.

Nontoxic and Also Inexpensive

Seeds for sprouts can be stored thirty to sixty years in a clean dry place. Sprouts are economical; for example five tablespoons of alfalfa seeds, which cost only 25 cents, will make a pound of alfalfa sprouts after four days of sprouting.

What Sprouts Have to Offer

- 100 percent organic, no pesticides or chemicals
- A high source of the enzymes that are needed to utilize foods
- A good source of antioxidant enzymes
- A concentrated source of antioxidant vitamins A, C, and E
- A good source of protein and minerals
- A source of chlorophyll to detoxify and enhance immunity
- The freshness of freshly grown food—the "live food factor"
- Low in calories and high in fiber
- You don't need a "green thumb," just soak and rinse twice daily

Sprouting Directions

Equipment:
- A wide-mouth sprouting jar
- Cheesecloth and elastic or plastic screening
- Or purchase a sprouting jar with screen cover
- Or purchase a tray type sprouter with cover
- Organic seeds

Directions:
- Purchase organic seeds
- Rinse the seeds with distilled, filtered, or spring water
- Put the seeds in the sprouting jar or tray and rinse well with clean water
- Drain
- Let jar rest at an angle so water drains out—cover with a cloth

- Rinse well twice daily—if foam appears in jar rinse till it is gone
- After sprouting time is up remove hulls by putting all the sprouts into a large pot and sifting out the sprouts leaving the hulls
- Cover and store in the refrigerator; will keep 5–7 days

Key Points:
- Remember to rinse thoroughly 2–3 times in 24-hour period
- Keep the sprouts moist, not wet
- Don't let them be overcrowded—they need to breathe
- Keep them covered, no light, until the last day of sprouting
- Then put them in indirect sunlight to develop chlorophyll

Sprout Recipe Ideas

Add to tossed salads
Use as a side dish with every meal
Add to coleslaw
Add to sautéed onions
Mix with fried rice as it cools
Create an open-face sandwich
Blend in vegetable juices

Sprouting Chart

TYPE OF SEED	AMOUNT OF SEEDS	YIELD	SOAK (IN HOURS)	RINSE (PER DAY)	HARVEST (IN DAYS)
adzuki bean	½ cup	2 cups	12	2–3	5–6
alfalfa	2 tablespoons	1 quart	4–6	2–3	4
garbanzo bean	1 cup	3 cups	12	2–3	3–4
lentil	1 cup	6 cups	8–12	2–3	3–4
mung bean	1 cup	4 cups	12	2–3	3–4
sunflower	1 cup	3 cups	12	2–3	3

Part IV

RESOURCES: A HANDY GUIDE FOR BOOKS AND MATERIALS

"Nature heals, but sometimes it needs a helping hand."
—*Bernard Jensen*

RESOURCES FOR CHAPTER 3: FOOD

Articles on Food

In addition to articles in the popular press, there are more than 500 articles in medical journals on free radicals. To read them you can go to a medical library (this usually requires some permission), or you can ask for a computer readout from the National Library of Medicine Medlars database, which contains the article title and a summary. One source for this is from:

Life Services
    MEDLARS Service
    (800) 542-3230
    Prices are from $20 to $40.

"The Possible Role of Free Radical Reactions in
Carcinogenesis"
H.B. Demopoulos et al.
Journal of Environmental Pathology and Toxicology,
1980, pp. 273–303

"The Development of Secondary Pathology with Free
Radicals: Reactions as a Threshold Mechanism"
H.B. Demopoulos et al.
Journal of American Col. Toxicology, 1983, pp. 173–84

"Oxygen Free Radicals Linked to Many Diseases"
J.L. Marx
Science, Jan. 30, 1987, pp. 249–531

"Role of Free Radical in Mutation, Cancer, Aging and the
Maintenance of Life"
Radiation Research 16:753–64, 1962

"Natural Chemicals Now Called Major Cause of Disease"
Jane Brody
New York Times, April 26, 1988

"Free Radical"
Natalie Angier
New York Times Magazine, April 25, 1993, p. 62

"Role of Free Radicals in Mutation, Cancer, Aging and the
Maintenance of Life"
Denham Harman
Radiation Research 16:753–54, 1962

"Free Radical Theory of Aging"
Denham Harman
Journal of Gerontology, Oct. 23, 1968

"Free Radical Theory of Aging: Nutritional Implications"
Denham Harman
AGE 1:145–52, 1978

"Free Radicals in Biological Systems"
W.A. Pryor
Scientific American, August 1970

"Free Radicals in Medicine: Chemical Nature and Biologic Reactions"
P.A. Southern and G. Powis
Mayo Clinic Proceedings 63:390–408, 1988

"Oxygen-Derived Free Radicals: Pathophysiology and Implications"
Mark Hitt, DVM
Compendium Small Animal, Vol. 10, No. 8, 1988, pp. 939–46

"Free Radical Biology: Xenobiotics, Cancer and Aging"
W.A. Pryor
New York Academy of Sciences Annals, Vol. 393, 1982, pp. 1–22

"Oxygen Poisoning and X-Irradiation: A Mechanism in Common"
R. Gerschman et al.
Science 119, 623 1954

"The New Scoop on Vitamins"
Time, April 6, 1992

"Vitamin C Intake and Mortality Among a Sample of the United States Population"
Enstrom et al.
Epidemiology 3:194–202, 1992

"Antioxidant Vitamins and Beta Carotene in Disease
Prevention"
The American Journal of Clinical Nutrition Proceedings
of a conference held in London, Oct. 2–4, 1989,
Supplement to Vol. 53, No. 1, January 1991

"Ascorbic Acid: Biologic Functions and Relation to
Cancer"
The American Journal of Clinical Nutrition Proceedings
of a conference held at the National Institutes of Health,
Bethesda, MD, Sept. 10–12, 1990, Supplement to Vol.
54, No. 6, December 1991

"Systemic Protection Against Radiation: Effect of an
Elemental Diet on Hematopoietic and Immunological
Systems in the Rat"
R. Pageau et al.
Radiation Research 62:357–63, 1975

"Effect of Dietary Calcium and Phosphorus Levels on Body
Burden of Ingested Radiostrontium"
H. Wasserman and C. Comar
*Society for Experimental Biology and Medicine
Proceedings* 103:124, 1960

"Vegetables, Fruit and Cancer"
K.A. Steinmetz and J.D. Potter
Cancer Causes and Control 2:427–42, 1991

"Glutathione in Foods Listed in National Cancer Institute
Health Habits and History of Food Questionnaire"
D.P. Jones et al.
Nutrition and Cancer 17:57–75, 1992

"Coronary Heart Disease Mortality Among Seventh Day
Adventists with Differing Dietary Habits"
R. Phillips
Abstract, American Public Health Association Meeting,
Chicago, Nov. 16–20, 1975

"Bowman-Birk Soybean Protease Inhibitor as an
Anticarcinogen"
J. Yavelow et al.
Cancer Research 43:2454–59, May 1983

"Relationship of Soybean Paste Soup Intake to Gastric
Cancer Risk"
T. Hirayama
Nutrition and Cancer 3:223–33, 1981

"Vitamin E Protects Against Free Radical Damage in Lipid
Environments"
R. Dean et al.
Bioc. Biop. R. 148:1277–82, 1987

"Antioxidants in Nutritional Medicine: Tocopheral,
Selenium and Glutathione"
J. Bland
In *Yearbook of Nutritional Medicine*, 1984–1985, ed. J.
Bland, Keats Publishing, 1985, pp. 213–37

"Nutritional Influence on Cellular Antioxidant Defense
Systems"
C. Chow
American Journal of Clinical Nutrition 32:1066, 1979

"Severe Impairment of Antioxidant System in Human
Hepatoma"
R. Corrocher et al.
Cancer 58:1658–62, 1986

"Ascorbic Acid Protects Lipids in Human Plasma and Low-Density Pipoprotein Against Oxidative Damage"
Balz Frei
American Journal of Clinical Nutrition 54:1113–18, 1991

"Role of Beta Carotene in Disease Prevention with Special Reference to Cancer"
V.N. Singh
Lipid-Soluble Antioxidants Biochemistry of Clinical Applications 208–27, 1992

"Mechanisms of Action of Biological Antioxidants"
N.I. Krinsky et al.
Proceedings for the Society for Experimental Biology 200:248–54, 1992

"Free Radical Antioxidants and Human Disease"
B. Halliwell et al.
Journal of Laboratory and Clinical Medicine 119:598–620, June 1992

"Selenium and Vitamins A, E and C: Nutrients with Cancer Prevention Properties"
R.R. Watson and T.K. Leonard
Journal of the American Dietetic Association 86:505–10, 1986

"Vitamin E and Autoxidation"
G.A. Fritsma
American Journal of Medical Technology 49:453–56, 1983

"Nutrition and Cancer: A Review with Emphasis on the Role of Vitamins C and E and Selenium"
P.M. Newberne and V. Saphakarn
Nutrition and Cancer 5:107–19, 1983

"Flavonoids Are Scavengers of Superoxide Anion"
J. Robak
Biochemical Pharmacological 37:2489–92, 1988

"Increased Green and Yellow Vegetables Intake and Lowered Cancer Deaths in an Elderly Population"
G.A. Colditz
American Journal of Clinical Nutrition 41(1):32–36, 1985

"Antitoxic Effects of Plant Fiber"
B.H. Ershoff
American Journal of Clinical Nutrition 27:1395, 1974

"The Influence of pH on the Survival After X-irradiation of Cultured Malignant Cells"
J. Haveman
International Journal of Radiation Biology 37:201–5, 1980

"Protease Inhibitors Suppress Radiation Induced Malignant Transformation in Vitro"
A. Kennedy and J. Little
Nature 276:825–26, 1978

"Effect of Brussel Sprouts and Cabbage on Drug Conjugation in Humans"
E.J. Pantuck et al.
Clinical Pharmacology and Therapeutics 35:161–69, 1984

"Antitumor Effect of Seaweed"
Y.I. Suzuki et al.
Chemotherapy 28(2):165–70, 1980

''Dietary Constituents Altering the Responses to Chemical
Carcinogens''
Lee Wattenberg et al.
*Federation of American Societies for Experimental
Biology Proceedings* 35:1327–31, 1976

''Coronary Heart Disease: Differing Dietary Habits''
R. Phillips
American Journal of Clinical Nutrition 31:181, 1978

''Traditional Diet and Food Preferences of Australian
Aboriginal Hunter-Gatherers''
Kerin O'Dea
*Philosophical Transactions of the Royal Society of
London* 334:223–41, 1991
For a copy of this article write:
Kerin O'Dea
Department of Human Nutrition
Deakin University
Geelong, Victoria 3217
Australia

''Eating Low on the Food Chain: For the Planet's Sake''
Hannah Holmes
Garbage, Jan.–Feb. 1992, pp. 32–37

''Relationship Between Radiocesium Contamination of Beef
and Milk''
G. Lacourley
Health Physics 21:793–802, 1971

''Chlorine in Drinking Water Causes Heart Attacks''
J.M. Quinlan
Cancer and Premature Aging, 1987 pp. 2–4

"Residue of Chemicals in Meat Leads to a Debate on
  Hazards"
  New York Times, March 15, 1983, p. 1

"Projected Dose Commitment from Fallout Contamination
  in Milk Resulting from the 1976 Chinese Atmospheric
  Nuclear Weapons Test"
  R.E. Simpson et al.
  Health Physics 40:741–43, May 1981

"Mutagens and Carcinogens in Foods"
  T. Sugimura and S. Sato
  Cancer Research 43:2415, 1983

"The Cs-137 Content of Beef from Dairy and Feedlot
  Cattle"
  G.M. Ward
  Health Physics 21:95–100, 1965

"PCB Levels Soar in Hudson Fish"
  Newsday, March 2, 1993

"Dietary Constituents Altering the Response to Chemical
  Carcinogens"
  Wattenberg et al.
  Federation Proceedings 35:1327–31, 1976

"Experimental Evidence for the Nutritional Superiority of
  Foods Grown with Organic Fertilization"
  Gar Hildenbrand
  Healing Newsletter, Vol. 5, No. 2, 1989

"Quality of Plants"
  Werner Schuphan
  Pl.Fds. Hum. Nutr. 23:4:333–58, 1974

"Organic Foods"
Ginia Bellafante
Garbage, Nov.–Dec. 1989

"A Trace of Pesticide, an Accepted Risk"
New York Times, "Week in Review," Feb. 7, 1993

"Epidemiological Correlations Between Diet and Cancer
Frequency"
P. Correa
Cancer Research 41:3685–90, 1981

"Dieldren Poisoning of Chickens During Severe Dietary
Restriction"
K.L. Davison et al.
Bulletin of Environmental Contamination and Toxicology
5:493–501, 1970

"Conditions for Inhibiting and Enhancing Effects of the
Protease Inhibitor on X-ray Induced Neoplastic
Formation"
C. Borek et al.
National Academy of Sciences of the United States
Biological Sciences Proceedings 76:1800–1903, 1979

Books on Food

Oxygen and Oxy-Radicals in Chemistry and Biology
M. Rogers and E. Powers
Academic Press, 1981

Life Extension
Durk Pearson and Sandy Shaw
Warner Books, 1982
The first popular book on the subject of free radicals and
how they affect health, and aging in particular.

May All Be Fed: Diet for a New World
　John Robbins
　William Morrow, 1992
　(800) 645-0555

Diet for a New America
　John Robbins
　Stillpoint Publishing, 1987
　(800) 645-0555

One Peaceful World
　Michio Kushi, 1987
　$17.95 plus $2 s&h to:
　One Peaceful World
　Box 10
　Becket, MA 11223
　This book is *must* reading.

The Macrobiotic Diet
　Michio and Aveline Kushi, 1991
　$17.00 plus $2 s&h to:
　One Peaceful World
　Box 10
　Becket, MA 11223

Conscious Eating
　Gabriel Cousens
　Vision Books, Santa Rosa, CA
　Comprehensive work on the role of food in your life.

The Cure Is in the Kitchen
　Sherry Rogers, M.D.
　Prestige Publishing, 1991
　(800) 846-ONUS
　$14.95 plus $3 s&h

Tired or Toxic?
Sherry Rogers, M.D.
Prestige Publishing, 1990
(800) 846-ONUS
$17.95 plus $3 s&h

Enzyme Nutrition
Edward Howell, M.D.
Avery Publishing Group, 1985
(800) 548-5757

Foods That Heal
Bernard Jensen
Avery Publishing Group, 1990
(800) 548-5757

Be Your Own Doctor: A Positive Guide to Natural Living
Ann Wigmore
Avery Publishing Group, 1983
(800) 548-5757

Fit for Life
Harvey and Marilyn Diamond
Warner Books, 1987

Spiritual Nutrition and the Rainbow Diet
Gabriel Cousens
Cassandra Press, 1986
A thoughtful book expanding the topic of food.

Antioxidant Adaptation: Its Role in Free Radical Pathology
S.A. Levine with P.M. Kidd
Allergy Research Group, San Leandro, CA, 1985

The Permanent Weight Loss Manual
Nathan Pritikin
Bantam, 1982

Oxidative Stress: Oxidants and Antioxidants
H. Sies
Academic Press, 1991

*Nutrition and Environmental Health: The Influence of
Nutritional Status on Pollutant Toxicity and
Carinogenicity*
Edward James Calbrese
John Wiley & Sons, 1980

Diet for a Small Planet
Frances Moore Lappé
10th anniversary edition, Ballantine Books, 1982

Diet for the Atomic Age
Sara Shannon
Avery, 1987

Beyond Beef: The Rise and Fall of the Cattle Culture
Jeremy Rifkin
Dutton, 1992

*The Changing American Diet: A Chronicle of Eating Habits
from 1910–1980*
L. Brewster and M. Jacobson
Center for Science in the Public Interest, Washington,
DC, 1983

*Radiation Exposure to the Public from Radioactive
Emissions of Nuclear Power Stations*
B. Franke et al.
Institute for Energy and Environmental Research (IFEU),
Heidelberg, West Germany. Translated by the NRC, 1980

*Cesium from the Environment to Man: Metabolism and
Dose*
E.A. Martell
NCRP Report No. 52 National Council on Radiation
Protection and Measurements, Washington, DC, 1977

Strontium Metabolism in Man
J. Lenihan, ed.
Academic Press, 1967

Nutritive Value of American Foods in Common Units
Agriculture Handbook No. 456, U.S. Dept. of
Agriculture 1987

*A Critical Review of Biological Accumulation
Discrimination, and Uptake of Radionuclides Important to
Waste Management Practices, 1943–1971*
K.R. Price
U.S. Dept. of Agriculture, 1971

Secrets of the Soil
Peter Tompkins and Christopher Bird
Harper & Row, 1989

Environmental Poisons in Our Food
Gordon J. Millichap
PNB Publishers (Box 11391, Chicago IL 60611), 1993

The Paleolithic Prescription
Boyd Eaton and Marjorie Shostak
Harper & Row, 1988

Nagasaki 1945
Tatsuichiro Akizuki
Quartet Books, 1981

*The Book of Macrobiotics: The Universal Way of Health
and Happiness*
Michio Kushi
Japan Publications, 1977

Cookbooks
The phone numbers listed below are for ordering the books.

Natural Foods Cookbook
Mary Estella
Japan Publications, 1985

Complete Guide to Macrobiotic Cooking
Aveline Kushi and Alex Jack
Japan Publications, 1985

The Book of Tofu
William Shurtleff and Akiko Aoyagi
Ballantine Books, 1976

The Book of Miso
William Shurtleff and Akiko Aoyagi
Ballantine Books, 1976

The Deaf Smith Country Cookbook
Marjorie Win Ford
Avery Publishing Group, 1991
(800) 548-5757

The Macrobiotic Cancer Prevention Cookbook
Aveline Kushi and Wendy Esko
Avery Publishing Group, 1988
(800) 548-5757

Whole Meals
Marcea Weber
Avery Publishing Group, 1988
(800) 548-5757

The TVP Cookbook
Dorothy Bates
The Book Publishing Company, 1991
(800) 695-2241
$6.95 plus $1.50 s&h.

The New Farm Vegetarian Cookbook
Louise Hagler
The Book Publishing Company, 1991
(800) 695-2241

Macrobiotic Cooking
Aveline Kushi with Alex Jack
Warner Books, 1975

The American Vegetarian Cookbook
Marilyn Diamond, 1992
(800) 435-9610

The New Laurel's Kitchen
Laurel Robertson, 1992
(800) 435-9610

Ecological Cooking: Recipes to Save the Planet
Joanne Stepaniank and Kathy Hecker
The Book Publishing Company, 1992
(800) 695-2241
$10.95 plus $1.50 s&h.

Sprout for the Love of Everybody
Viktoras Kulvinskas
A compact booklet on sprouting.

Love Your Body
  Viktoras Kulvinskas
  Contains 200 recipes using raw foods.
  The above two books available from:
  21st Century Publications
  (800) 593-2665

*No More Allergies: Identifying and Eliminating Allergies
  and Sensitivity Reactions to Everything in Your
  Environment*
  Gary Null
  Villard Books, 1992
  A plan, including recipes, for treating food allergies and
  chemical sensitivities and a listing of over 250
  environmentally oriented health care practitioners.

Catalogue for Books on Health
Aurora Book Companions
  Box 5852
  Denver, CO 80217
  The world's largest distributor of health-related books.
  Their catalogue lists both by subject and by author.

Books on Candida
Coping with Candida Cookbook
  Sally Rockwell
  (800) 227-2627
  Low-carbohydrate menus with no milk, eggs, yeast, fruit,
  or sugar.

The Yeast Connection
  William Crook, M.D.
  (800) 287-2687
  Tells how to overcome the chronic health problems
  related to *Candida albicans* infections.

The Yeast Connection Cookbook
William Crook, M.D.
(800) 227-2627
Over 200 recipes focusing on the foods that will help
overcome candida.

The Silent Menace
Dorothy Senerchia
Strawberry Hill Press, 1990
Tells how to live with candida and includes 70 pages of
recipes by a woman who suffered from the ''20th century
epidemic.''

Resources for Natural and Organic Foods
Living Farms
Box 50
Tracy, MN 56175
(800) 533-5320
They have organic grains. Call for complete product list.
They ship nationwide.

Natural Way Mills, Inc.
Rte. 2, Box 37
Middle River, MN 56737
(218) 222-3677
They have whole grains and flours. Call for complete
product list. They ship nationwide.

Maine Seaweed Company
P.O. Box 57
Steuben, ME 04680
(207) 546-2875
You can find Maine seaweed in your health store or buy
directly from them, for example, the ''family pack,'' a
selected mix of five types of seaweeds for $45 (s&h

included). They also take apprentices during the harvest season of May-June.

Mountain Ark
120 South East Avenue
Fayetteville, AR 72701
(800) 643-8900
A complete natural food store. Call for catalogue.

Gold Mine Natural Food Company
1947 30th Street
San Diego, CA 92102
(800) 475-FOOD
Macrobiotic, organic foods and kitchen and other home products. They feature a "macro sampler kit" for $99.95 that includes rice, grains, beans, seeds, sea vegetables, sesame oil, tea, and more. A good way to stock up with the basics.

Diamond Organics
Freedom, CA
(800) 922-2396
They feature organically grown vegetables delivered overnight to you anywhere in the United States. Call for catalogue.

The Mushroom People
P.O. Box 220
Summertown, TN 38483-0090
They have a kit for making tempeh with directions, $4. Kit which makes six pounds of tempeh, $15. Send for their catalogue, which includes mushrooms, other foods, and books published by The Farm.

Sprouts
Life Sprouts
>P.O. Box 150
>Paradies, UT 84328-0150
>(800) 241-1516
>They sell a sprouter called the Sprout Master, and they sell organic sprouting seeds.

Natural Food Systems
>P.O. Box 1028
>Pagosa Springs, CO 81147
>(800) 874-2733
>They sell a sprouter and organic seeds and beans. They also have a long-term seed- and bean-storage program.

The Sprout House
>P.O. Box 1100
>Great Barrington, MA 01230
>(413) 528-5200
>They have various sprouters and sprouting kits, and sell seeds in bulk. A newsletter is $10 for 32 issues yearly. An audiocassette on indoor gardening is $9.

Reading on Sprouts
Sprout for the Love of Everybody
>Viktoras Kulvinskas
>21st Century Publications, 1978

Recipes for Life
>Dr. Ann Wigmore
>Hippocrates Press, 1985

Survival into the 21st Century
>Viktoras Kulvinskas
>21st Century Publications, 1975

Spiritual Nutrition and the Rainbow Diet
Gabriel Cousens
Cassandra Press, 1986

Organizations

EarthSave
P.O. Box 68
Santa Cruz, CA 95063-0068
(800) DNA-DOIT
An organization founded by John Robbins focusing on health and the environment. They have a newsletter and a catalogue of books and some products.

Northeast Center for Environmental Medicine
P.O. Box 3161
Syracuse, NY 13220
(315 455-7862
Founded by Dr. Sherry Rogers to share information about environmental illness and identify environmental triggers that cause many diseases. Their health letter is $15 a year (4 issues).

North American Vegetarian Society
P.O. Box 72
Dolgeville, NY 13329
(518) 568-7970

One Peaceful World
Box 10
Becket, MA 01223
(413) 623-2322
An international society of people devoted to the realization of one healthy, peaceful world. The OPW newsletter is included with membership.

Residential Health Retreats
Kushi Institute of the Berkshires
P.O. Box 7
Becket, MA 01223
(413) 623-5742
Residential seminars. The seven-day macrobiotic residential seminar includes cooking classes, lectures on diet, shiatsu, and more. Tuition includes all of the above on a 600 acre estate of forests, meadows, and streams.

Sage Mountain Herb Center
P.O. Box 420
East Barre, VT 05649
(802) 479-9825
Workshops in herbalism and earth awareness on 500 wilderness acres.

Vega Study Center
1511 Robinson Street
Oroville, CA 95965
Send for brochure of their weekends, weeks, and other courses. Includes cooking and special healing stays.

Hippocrates Health Institute
1443 Palmdale Court
West Palm Beach, FL 33411
(800) 842-2125
Health building stays featuring wheat grass, juices, and raw food in the healing sunshine.

Holistic Health Directory
P.O. Box 53275
Boulder, CO 80321-3275
(800) 782-7006

Published by the *New Age Journal*, the *Holistic Health Directory* is a good listing of resources for healing modalities. $5.95.

Ann Wigmore Institute
P.O. Box 429
Rincón, Puerto Rico 00677
(809) 868-6307
Ann Wigmore is the founder of the living foods lifestyle and developer of wheatgrass therapy. A unique and simple healing routine based on raw foods.

Health Education

Gulliver's Learning Center
150 West 53rd Street, Suite 37E
New York, NY
(212) 541-5433
Offers a series of lectures on food and health philosophy.

Natural Gourmet Cooking School
48 West 21st Street
New York, NY 10010
(212) 645-5170
A variety of practical cooking courses, also a chef's training program.

Kushi Institute
P.O. Box 1100
Brookline Village, MA 02147
(413) 623-5742
Residential cooking and way-of-life classes. Also a summer retreat-conference in beautiful New England.

▲

"Since the 1930's, 7 million family farmers have lost their land. . . . The backbone of our country is broken. The farmers who used to care for the land and feed our families are now standing in unemployment lines. Everyone who wants healthful food must make a decision to do something."
—WILLIE NELSON, Letter to the Editor, *USA Today*, April 23, 1993

▲

Farming

For information on the plight of the farmer:

Torn from the Land (videotape)
Life and Health Publications
465 N.E. 181 Street, Suite 16
Portland, OR 97230
$26.00 including s&h

Basic Formula to Create Community Supported Agriculture
Robyn VanEn
Indian Line Farm RR3
Box 85
Great Barrington, MA 01230
Contains information on how to become a shareholder in a farm—or to turn your farm into a community-supported project. Available for $10.

Kusa Research Foundation
P.O. Box 761
Ojai, CA 93024
A consumer information resource for small-scale production of traditional edible seedcrops. This group

feels that humans have a genetic attunement for food that is produced small-scale, and that this should be taught in schools. Send $1 and a large-size SASE for information about membership.

Two Organizations Focusing on Agriculture
CSA Committee for Sustainable Agriculture
P.O. Box 1300
Colfax, CA 95713
(916) 346-2777

IAA Institute of Alternative Agriculture
9200 Edmonton Road #117
Greenbelt, MD
(301) 441-8777

A Solar Greenhouse
The Biodome™ is an energy-efficient way to have wholesome, fresh produce accessible year-round. It is a solar greenhouse developed at the Windstar Foundation of Snowmass, Colorado, and is based on the principles of Buckminster Fuller. Biodomes are well suited for harsh climates and will extend a seasonal backyard or community garden into a year-round gardening experience. They are in a diameter of 15, 27, 36, and 56 feet. It is solar-heated and cooled and contains fish tanks that produce fish for protein, and also serve as cooling in summer and heating in winter.

Biodome
Windstar Foundation
2317 Snowmass Creek Road
Snowmass, CO 81654
(303) 927-4777

Sources for Seeds

Ten companies own 80 percent of the world's seed market, so it is important to have your own garden and your own seeds.

Seeds of Change
621 Old Santa Fe Trail
Santa Fe, NM 87501
(505) 983-8956
They specialize in certified organic seeds. Send $3 for a catalogue. They have a consulting service on sustainable organic farming and occasional conferences in New Mexico. Great resource!

The Seed Savers Exchange
Route 3
Box 239
Decorah, IA 52101
For information on saving your seeds from year to year and exchanging them, enclose $1 for brochure.

Johnny's Selected Seeds
Foss Hill Road
Albion, ME 04910

Abundant Life Seed Foundation
P.O. Box 772
Port Townsend, WA 98368

Shepherd's Garden Seeds
30 Irene Street
Torrington, CT 06790
(203) 482-3638
A catalogue of seeds for vegetables, herbs, and flowers, specializing in selections from European, Japanese, and Chinese seed houses. They have some special varieties of

the antioxidant vegetables such as kale, watercress, and cabbage; also a packet of eight easy-to-grow vegetables and flowers for children with an explanatory brochure called "A Special Garden for Children."

Residential Gardening

Findhorn Foundation
Accommodation Secretary
Cluny Hill College
Forres, IV36 ORO
Scotland
Findhorn Foundation is a community of around 150 people with some 4,000 paying guests per year who absorb the foundation's unique quality of relationship to the land and nature.

Agroecology Program
University of California, Santa Cruz
Santa Cruz, CA 95064
(408) 459-4140
Graduate and undergraduate courses and public education programs.

Books on Gardening and Farming

Seeds of Change: The Living Treasure
The Seeds of Change Group
Harper, San Francisco 1993
(505) 438-8080
Includes interviews with master organic gardeners and inspired seed collectors with stunning photos of enchanted gardens.

The New Organic Growers Four Seasons Harvest: How to Harvest Fresh Organic Vegetables from Your Home Garden All Year Long
Eliot Coleman
Chelsea Green Publishing Company, 1992

Super Nutrition Gardening
William Peavy
Avery Publishing Group, 1992
(800) 548-5757

Encyclopedia of Organic Gardening
Rodale Press, 1992

Secrets of the Soil
Peter Tompkins and Christopher Bird
Harper & Row, 1989
Must reading.

For information on bio-dynamic gardening:
Bio-Dynamic Farming and Gardening Association
P.O. Box 550
Kimberton, PA 19442
(215) 935-7797

For information on soil remineralization:
Soil Remineralization
Joanna Camp
152 South Street
Northampton, MA 01060

Resource for books by Rudolph Steiner and about farming:
Anthroposophic Press
Bells' Pond, Star Route
Hudson, NY 12534
(518) 851-2054

A catalogue book house on organic gardening:
Ag Access
P.O. Box 2008
Davis, CA 95617

The Findhorn Garden
by the Findhorn Community
Foreword by William Irwin Thompson
Harper Colophon Books, 1968

*Supernutrition Gardening: How to Grow Your Own
Powercharged Foods*
William Peavy and Warren Peavy
Avery Publishing Group, 1993
(800) 548-5757

Soil-Testing Services

For soil-testing services with specific recommendations for organic gardeners:

Timberleaf Farm
5569 State Street
Albany, OH 45710
(614) 698-3681

Necessary Trading Company
One Nature's Way
New Castle, VA 24127
(703) 864-5103

For Information on Soil Remineralization
Remineralize the Earth
152 South Street
Northampton, MA 01061

For Information on Organic Certification Standards
Organic Crop Improvement Association
  (513) 592-4983

CSA Directory (Committee for Sustainable Agriculture)
  c/o WTIG
  818 Connecticut Avenue, N.W.
  Suite 800
  Washington, DC 20006
  You can buy a share in a community-supported farm by
  making a payment before the growing season. You will
  receive fresh organic vegetables and fruits throughout the
  growing season. There are about 200 such farms around
  the country. Most are organic but check first before you
  buy your share.

RESOURCES FOR CHAPTER 4:
SUPPLEMENTS

Popular Books with Discussion of Free Radicals and Antioxidants

Formula for Life
Eberhard and Phyllis Kronhausen
William Morrow, 1989

Life Extension
Durk Pearson and Sandy Shaw
Warner Books, 1982

Reverse the Aging Process Naturally
Gary Null
Villard Books, 1993

364 GOOD HEALTH IN A TOXIC WORLD

Maximum Immunity
Michael Weiner
Houghton Mifflin, 1989

Nutritional Healing
James and Phyllis Balch
Avery Publishing Group, 1990
(800) 548-5757

Related Books

Antioxidant Adaptation: Its Role in Free Radical Pathology
Stephen Levine and P.M. Kidd
Allergy Research Group, 1985
This comprehensive books is available for $40 plus $5 postage from:
Allergy Research Group
P.O. Box 489
San Leandro, CA 94577
(510) 569-9064

Free Radicals in Biology and Medicine, 2nd edition
B. Hallwell and J.M.C. Gyteridge
Clarendon Press, Oxford, 1989

Biochemical Individuality
Roger Williams, M.D.
University of Texas Press, Austin, 1956

Oxidative Stress: Oxidants and Antioxidants
H. Sies
Academic Press, 1991

Oxy-Radicals and Their Scavenging Systems
G. Cohen and R. Greenwald, eds.
Vol. 1, pp. 1–399
Elsevier Biochemical, NY, 1983

Absorption Study with SOD/CAT
P.R. Rotschild
University Labs Press, 1215 Center Street
Honolulu, HI 96828

Keats Publishing
27 Pine Street
Box 876
New Canaan, CT 06840
Health booklets by experts on specific topics, including herbs, antioxidants, supplements, and foods, mostly priced around $2.25

The Colon Health Handbook
Robert Gray
Emerald Publishing, Dept. AE-1
Box 11830
Reno, NV 89510
$6.95 for a classic book discussing how the condition of the colon is interconnected with the health of the entire body and suggestions for improvement.

Oxygen Therapies
Ed McCabe
Energy Publications
available from:
The Family News
777 South State Road 7, #51
Margate, FL 33068
(800) 284-6263
Unique book on the benefits of oxygenation. Virus and bacteria cannot live in oxygen.

Options: The Alternative Cancer Therapy Book
  Richard Walters
  Avery Publishing Group 1993
  (800) 548-5757
  Therapeutic options and resources.

Articles on Antioxidants

To obtain copies of medical journals

There are more than 3,000 orthodox biomedical and health journals regularly published. The National Library of Medicine places abstracts of every article from every journal on computer databases and this is available to everyone. The information contains the latest in conventional treatments and discussions of diseases. Also in the database is every article on prevention, nutrition, and supplements found in mainstream medical journals. Seven regional libraries located at major medical colleges can help you with a search or article request. Many public libraries have access to MEDLARS databases and can perform searches for a cost of between $10 and $50.

For more information:
MEDLARS
  National Library of Medicine
  8600 Rockville Place
  Bethesda, MD 20894
  (800) 638-8480
  FAX (301) 496-0822
  Another source for a computer readout:

Life Services
  Medlars Service
  (800) 542-3230
  Prices are from $20 to $40.

Those who are interested in reading any of the articles in this book may go in person to:

New York Academy of Medicine
2 East 103rd Street
New York, NY 10029
(212) 876-8200
FAX (212) 722-7650
Or you may order copies of articles by mail from them for a fee of $8 per article prepaid. The volume, date, and page numbers should be included. Orders will be processed within five days. For quicker service, articles may be faxed the next day for a fee of $16 per article.

To Obtain Copies of Articles on Therapeutic Benefits of Plants

There are about 200 journals on therapeutic benefits of plants and many books published annually. The NAPRAL-ERT, which stands for Natural Products Alert, is a computer database of the scientific articles and books on the constituents and pharmacology of plants. There is a fee of $10 for each search, and any article longer than three pages is 50 cents per page.

NAPRALERT
Program for Collaborative Research in the Pharmaceutical Sciences
College of Pharmacy
University of Illinois at Chicago
P O Box 6998
Chicago, IL 60680
(312) 996-7523

Articles on Supplements

"Historical Perspective: Antioxidants, Nutrition and Evolution (Vitamin, A, Vitamin E, Vitamin C, Selenium)"
Thomas Jukes
Preventive Medicine 21:270–76, 1992

"Beta-Carotene and Vitamin A"
Thomas Edes
The Nutrition Report 10:9, Feb. 1992

"The Role of Glutathione in Aging and Cancer"
John Richie
Experimental Gerontology 27:615–26, 1992

"Protective Role of Dietary Vitamin E on Oxidative Stress in Aging"
Mohsen Meydani
AGE 15:89–93, 1992
To ask for a reprint at no charge write to:
Mohsen Meydani, Ph.D.
Antioxidant Research Laboratory
USDA Human Nutrition Research Center on Aging at Tufts University
711 Washington Street
Boston, MA 02401

"Cellular Antioxidant Status in Human Immunodeficiency Virus Replication"
D. Baker
Nutrition Reviews 50:15–17, 1992
To ask for a reprint at no charge write to:
Nutrition Reviews
Springer-Verlag
175 Fifth Avenue
New York, NY 10010

"Glutathione Deficiency and Human Immunodeficiency
   Virus Infection"
   Frank Stall et al.
   Lancet, April 11, 1992

"Antioxidants in the Prevention of Human Atherosclerosis"
   Summary and Proceediings of the National Heart, Lung
   and Blood Institute
   Workshop, Sept. 1991
   Bethesda, MD
   Circulation 85:2388–94, June 1992
   To ask for a reprint write:
   Dr. Daniel Steinberg
   Division of Endocrinology 0613D
   University of California at San Diego
   Basic Science Building, Room 1080
   La Jolla, CA 92093

"Oxygen Radicals and Atherosclerosis"
   K.L. Carpenter et al.
   Klin Wochenschr 69:1039–45, 1991
   To order a reprint:
   Dr. K.L. Carpenter
   Department of Pathology
   University of Cambridge
   Cambridge CB21QP
   England

"Ascorbate: The Most Effective Antioxidant in Human
   Blood Plasma"
   B. Frei et al.
   Advances in Experimental and Medical Biology
   264:155–63, 1990

"Potential Clinical Applications for High-Dose Nutritional Antioxidants"
E.J. Crary
Medical Hypotheses 13:77–98, Jan. 1984

"A Review of Epidemiologic Evidence That Carotinoids Reduce Risk of Cancer"
R.G. Zeigler
Journal of Nutrition 119:116–22, 1989

"Regulation of Cellular Glutathione"
S.M. Deneke and B.L. Fanburg
American Journal of Physiology 257:163–73, 1989

"Scientific Basis for the Clinical Use of Superoxide Dismutase"
A. Petkau
Cancer Treatment Reviews 13:17–44, 1986

"Antioxidant Vitamins and Coronary Heart Disease"
D. Steinberg
New England Journal of Medicine 328:1487–89, 1993

"Oxidative Stress: Oxidants and Antioxidants"
A. Spector
In *The Lens and Oxidative Stress*, 1991, Chapter 19, pp. 529–58

"Effect of Exposure to Air Pollution on the Need for Antioxidant Vitamins"
Daniel Menzel
Beyond Deficiency: New Views on Function and Health Effects of Vitamins
New York Academy of Sciences, Feb. 9–12, 1992, Abstract 13

"Mechanisms of Action of Biological Antioxidants"
Norman Krinsky
Proceedings in the Society of Experimental Biology and Medicine 200:248–54, 1992

"Free Radicals, Antioxidants and Human Disease: Where Are We Now?"
B. Halliwell
Journal of Laboratory and Clinical Medicine
119:598–620, June 1992

"Antioxidant and Vitamin Supplementation: How Safe?"
N. Flodin
The Nutrition Report 10:25–32, April 1992

"Antioxidant Functions of Vitamins"
Helmut Sies
Beyond Deficiency: New Views on Function and Health Effects of Vitamins
New York Academy of Sciences, Feb. 9–12, 1992, Abstract 1

"The Superoxide Free Radical: Its Biochemistry and Pathophysiology"
J.M. McCord
Surgery 94:404–8, 1983

"Tocopherols, Carotenoids and the Glutathione System"
Helmut Sies
Lipid-Soluble Antioxidants: Biochemistry and Clinical Application, 160–65, 1992

"Selenium and Vitamins A, E, and C: Nutrients with Cancer Prevention Properties"
R.E. Watson and T.K. Leonard
Journal of American Dietetic Association 86:505–10, 1986

"Vitamin E and Autoxidation"
G.A. Fritsma
American Journal of Medical Technology 49:453–56,
1983

"Nutrition and Cancer: A Review with Emphasis on the
Role of Vitamins C and E and Selenium"
P.M. Newberne and V. Saphakarn
Nutrition and Cancer 5:107–119, 1983

"Vitamin E Protects Against Free Radical Damage in Lipid
Environments"
R. Dean et al.
Biochemistry Biophysical Research 148:1277–82, 1987

"Ascorbic Acid Protects Lipids in Human Plasma and Low-
Density Lipoprotein Against Oxidative Damage"
Balz Frei
American Journal of Clinical Nutrition 54:1113–18, 1991

"Vitamin C Intake and Mortality Among a Sample of the
United States Population"
Enstrom et al.
Epidemiology 3:194–202, 1992

"Antioxidant Vitamins and Beta Carotene in Disease
Prevention"
The American Journal of Clinical Nutrition
Proceedings of a conference held at the National Institutes
of Health, Bethesda, MD, Sept. 10–12, 1992
Supplement to Vol. 54, No. 6, December 1991

"Detoxifying, Radioprotective and Phagocyte-Enhancing
Effects of Garlic"
Benjamine Lau, M.D.
International Journal of Clinical Nutritional Review Vol.
19, No. 1, Jan. 1989

"Antiviral Activity of Alliu, Sativum (Garlic)"
N. Weber et al.
Abstracts Annual Meeting, American Society for
Microbiology 88:22, 1988

"Activation of Immuno-Responder Cells by the Protein
Fraction from Aged Garlic Extract"
Y. Hirao et al.
Phytotherapy Research 1:161–64, 1987

"Garlic Compounds Modulate Macrophage and T-
Lymphocyte Functions"
B. Lau et al.
Molecular Biotherapy, Vol. 3, June 1991, pp. 103–7

"Antitumor-Promoting Activity of Allixin, A Stress
Compound Produced by Garlic"
H. Nishino et al.
The Cancer Journal 3:20–24, Jan. 1990

"Nutrition: At the Crossroads"
Brian Liebovitz
Journal of Optimal Nutrition, 1992:1:69–83

The American Journal of Clinical Nutrition, January 1992
This 205-page special issue is entirely devoted to the
topic of antioxidant vitamins. The reports confirm the
causality of free radicals in degenerative diseases and the
fact that antioxidant nutrients can help alleviate this
damage. Available in a medical library or directly from
the journal. Supplements from the American Journal of
Clinical Nutrition can be obtained from:

AJCN Supplements
  9650 Rockville Pike, Room 3404
  Bethesda, MD
  (301) 530-7038
  Price is $25 plus s&h

"Vitamin E: Interactions with Free Radicals and Ascorbate"
  P. McCay
  Annual Review of Nutrition, 1985, pp. 323–40

"Aspects of the Structure, Function and Applications of
  Superoxide Dismutase"
  J.V. Bannister et al.
  Critical Reviews in Biochemistry, Vol. 22, 1987, pp.
  111–80

"The Antioxidant Role of Vitamin C"
  A. Bendich et al.
  Advances on Free Radical Biological Medicine, 1986, pp.
  419–44

"Beta Carotene: An Unusual Type of Lipid Antioxidant"
  G.W. Burton et al.
  Science, 1984, pp. 569–73

"Protective Roles of Minerals Against Free Radical
  Damage"
  J.F. Combs
  Nutrition, American Institute of Nutrition, 1987

"On the Quenching of Singlet Oxygen by Alpha-
  Tocopheral"
  S.R. Fahrenholtz et al.
  Photochemical Photobiological, 1974, pp. 505–9

"Plasma Levels of Antioxidant Vitamins in Relation to Ischaemic Heart Disease and Cancer"
L.F. Gey
American Journal of Clinical Nutrition, 1987, pp. 1368–77

"Superoxide Dismutase and Glutathione Peroxidase Activities in Erythrocytes as Indices of Oxygen Loading Disease: A Survey of 100 Cases"
L.L. Tho and J.K. Candlish
Biochemical Medicine and Metabolic Biology, 1987, pp. 74–80

"Superoxide Dismutase: Correlation with Life Span and Specific Metabolic Rate in Primate Species"
J. Tolmasoff et al.
Proceedings of the National Academy of Science, 1980, p. 2777

"Antioxidant Nutrients and Disease Prevention"
A.T. Diplock
American Journal of Clinical Nutrition, 1991, p. 190

Effect of Cell Guard on the Health of Children Following the Chernobyl Nuclear Accident
N.A. Gres and T.I. Polyakova
Radiation Medicine Research Institute
Ministry of Health, Republic of Belarus
(Cell Guard is an antioxidant enzyme formulated by Biotec.)

Newsletters

The Environmental Newsletter
Northeast Center for Environmental Medicine
P.O. Box 3638
Syracuse, NY 13220
(315) 455-7862
An excellent newsletter on all aspects of environmental
illness by a medical expert in this field, Dr. Sherry
Rogers. One year, $18. Published quarterly.

Clinical Pearls Health Letter
IT Services
3301 Alta Arden
Sacramento, CA
(800) 422-9887
(916) 488-1710
A health letter on nutrition and preventive medicine that
provides 25 to 30 summaries of medical journal articles
and includes some editorial commentary. Excellent for
health practitioners and the interested layperson. Ten
copies a year are $40.

Townsend Letter for Doctors
911 Tyler Street
Port Townsend, WA 98368-6541
An outstanding resource of current information.
Bimonthly. 1 year, $38.

HealthFacts
Center for Medical Consumers
237 Thompson Street
New York, NY 10012
(212) 674-7205
1 year, $21—12 issues. The Center for Medical
Consumers is a unique library for the health consumer.

Located in downtown NYC, it has up-to-date information on ailments, treatments, and options, with medical journals, health journals, and clippings organized by topic.

Journals

Journal of Optimal Nutrition (JON)
Subscription Department
2552 Regis Drive
Davis, CA 95616
(916) 756-3311
A journal focusing on the use of nutrients in prevention of disease and maintenance of optimum health. A quarterly peer-reviewed journal. $75 per year.

Explore
P.O. Box 1508
Mount Vernon, WA 98273
(206) 424-6025
A fine journal on alternative approaches to health. 6 issues, $59.

Resources for Supplements

Specialty Items
Blue-Green Algae
A resource for the nutrient-rich, wild, organic, free-radical-fighting food supplement, blue-green algae; and a special antioxidant enzyme formulation called Super Sprouts.
June Johns
(800) 775-8081 X2778

True Hart Nutrition, Inc.
(212) 966-5687
For flax oil, Essiac tea, and other items.

N.E.E.D.S. (National Ecological and Environmental
  Delivery System)
  527 Charles Avenue, Suite 12A
  Syracuse, NY 13209
  (800) 634-1380
  A fine selection of items for those with allergies, candida,
  environmental illness, CFS, and other conditions of
  compromised immunity. Ask for their catalogue.

The Buyers Club
  1187 Coast Village
  RD #1, 280
  Santa Barbara, CA 93108-2794
  (800) 366-6056
  Nutritional supplements at a special price.

Hickey Chemists
  888 Second Avenue
  New York, NY
  (212) 223-6333/(800) 724-5566
  One of the single best resources for a selection of quality
  supplements. Will mail anywhere.

Companies That Make Supplements

Most of these can be found in your health store, some
sell in wholesale for quantity purchases, and most provide
informational material.

A.C. Grace Company
  1100 Quit Man Road
  P.O. Box 570
  Big Sandy, TX 75755
  (903) 636-4368

Alacer Corporation
  14 Morgan
  Irvine, CA 92718
  (714) 951-9660
  Their product, Emergen-C, is a powdered vitamin C drink
  combined with some minerals in a handy individual
  packet. Good for after exercise instead of Gatorade.

Allergy Research Group
  400 Preda Street
  San Leandro, CA 94577
  (800) 545-9960
  Specially formulated products by Dr. Stephen Levine.
  Mainly sold through health practitioners. Descriptive
  catalogue available.

Biotec Food Corporation
  2639 South King Street #206
  Honolulu, HI 96826
  (800) 468-7578
  Unique antioxidant enzyme formulas that are enteric-
  coated so they can be utilized. Ask for an information
  packet.

Ecological Formulas
  106 "B" Shary Circle
  Concord, CA 94518
  (510) 827-2636/(800) 888-4585
  Thoughtfully formulated for the allergic or sensitive
  person and aimed toward building immunity

Country Life Vitamins
  180 Oser Avenue
  Hauppage, NY 11788
  (800) 645-5768
  Up-to-date formulations found in most health stores.

Eclectic Institute
  11231 S.E. Market Street
  Portland, OR 97216
  (800) 332-HERB
  Special freeze-dried herbal products and extracts, as well as vitamin formulas.

Freeda
  36 East 41st Street
  New York, NY 10017
  (800) 777-3737
  A family-run company that makes quality formulas.

KAL Healthway Vitamins
  P.O. Box 4023
  Woodland Hills, CA 91365
  (818) 340-3035
  A good line of products found in most health stores.

Klaire Laboratories
  1573 West Seminole
  San Marcos, CA 92069
  (619) 744-9680/(800) 533-7255
  A good line of products found in many health stores.

Kroeger Herb Products
  1122 Pearl Street
  Boulder, CO 80302
  (303) 443-0755
  A specialty line of herbs sensitively formulated by Hanna Kroeger.

Nature's Herbs
  P.O. Box 336
  Orem, UT 84663
  (800) 9-NATURE
  A fine selection of herbal products.

Solgar
  410 Ocean Avenue
  Lynbrook, N.Y. 11563
  (800) 645-2246
  A dependable company, their supplements found in most
  health stores.

Source Naturals
  23 Janus Way
  Scotts Valley, CA 95066
  (800) 777-5677
  Quality supplements.

Standard Process Laboratories
  12209 Locksley Lane, Suite 15
  Auburn, CA 95603
  (916) 888-1974/(800) 662-9134
  A special line of supplements using glandular substances
  and nutrients. Sold mostly through naturopathic doctors.

Twin Labs
  2120 Smithtown Avenue
  Ronkonkoma, NY 11779
  (800) 645-5626
  Extensive selection of formulations, many geared to
  fighting free radicals. Available in most health stores.

Wakunaga of America
  23501 Madero
  Mission Viejo, CA 92691
  (800) 544-5800/(800) 421-2998
  They make Kyolic, the odorless garlic, which is an
  antioxidant and premier detoxifier and immunity builder.

Yerba Prima
  P.O. Box 2569
  Oakland, CA 94614
  (800) 421-9972
  Herbal products and fiber colon cleansers.

Health Organizations

American Holistic Medical Association
  6932 Little River Turnpike
  Annandale, VA 22003

International Academy of Preventive Medicine
  10409 Town and County Way
  Houston, TX 77024

National Association of Naturopathic Physicians
  2613 North Stevens
  Tacoma, WA 98407

American Academy of Environmental Medicine
  109 West Olive Street
  Fort Collins, CO 80524

Foundation for the Advancement of Innovative Medicine
  2 Executive Boulevard
  Suffern, NY 10901
  (914) 268-FUND

Education on health care alternatives. They have two-day
symposiums twice a year in New York City. Very current
and insightful.

National Vaccination and Information Center
(703) 938-0342
Information on possible weakening effects of
vaccinations.

Vaccination Alternatives
(212) 870-5117
Guidance for thoughtful reconsideration of vaccinations.

Nutri-Cology
400 Pedra Street
San Leandro, CA 94577
(510) 639-4572
A partial nationwide list of physicians who treat candida.
Ask for a computerized list of doctors in your area. Give
your zip code.

The Cheney Clinic
10602 Park Road
Suite 234
Charlotte, NC 28210
(704) 542-7444
They specialize in the diagnosis and treatment of CFIDS
(chronic fatigue syndrome). Call for their information
pack if you are interested in an appointment.

Dr. Sherry Rogers
Box 2716
Syracuse, NY 13220
(315) 488-2856

Dr. Rogers specializes in environmental illness, chronic fatigue syndrome and other diseases of weakened immunity.

Health Tapes
FACT
Box 1242
Old Chelsea Station
New York, NY 19113
A variety of audiotapes on key health topics.

Database on Alternative Health
IBIS (The Interactive Body/Mind Information System)
Format Macintosh or IBM
IBIS is a database of information on alternative health containing a huge amount of data on 282 Western medical conditions, and syndromes from Chinese medicine. It has the ability to cross-reference therapies. It was created for alternative health care providers, but it could be fascinating for anyone interested in health. For an information packet send $2 to:
New Horizons
19 Exchange Street
Charleston, SC 29401
(800) 775-8081 ext. 2778

Books on Herbs
The New Age Herbalist
R. Mabey
Macmillan, 1988

Planetary Herbology
Michael Tierra
Lotus Press, 1988

*Potter's New Cyclopedia of Botanical Drugs and
Preparations*
Potter and Clarke, 1975

The Way of Herbs
Michael Tierra
Pocket Books, 1990

Back to Eden
Jethro Kloss
Woodbridge Press, 1972

School of Natural Healing
Dr. John Christopher
(801) 489-8787
A reference volume on herbs for the teacher or herbal
practitioner.

Inner Traditions International Press
One Park Street
Rochester, VT 05767
An excellent catalogue of books on botanicals and
medicine

Literature Research on Herbs
Herb Research Foundation
1007 Pearl Street, Ste. 200
Boulder, CO 80302
(303) 449-2265
fax (303) 449-7849
They have research and information on herbs, including
abstracts of major scientific articles on over 250 herbs,
and ethno-botanical studies.

Magazine
HerbalGram
    P.O. Box 201660
    Austin, TX 78720
    An excellent magazine on herbs and botanical medicine.

Video
Edible and Medicinal Herbs
    Wise Woman Herbals
    P.O. Box 328
    Gladstone, OR 97027
    VHS, 60 minutes, discusses over 20 plants. $39.95

Study Herbs
The School of Natural Healing
    Springville, UT 84663
    (800) 453-1406
    Founded by Dr. John Christopher 40 years ago. Offers a
    home study course and a master herbalist course on site.
    Ask for free brochure.

The Oregon School of Herbal Studies
    25031 Lavell Road
    Junction City, OR 97448
    (503) 998-3698
    They offer one-day, weekend, and four-month herbal
    courses.

Green Messenger Herbs
    P.O. Box U
    Hewitt, NJ 07421
    Apprenticeships. Send SASE for information.

Sources for Herbs
Christopher Family Herbals
  188 South Main
  Springville, UT 84663
  (801) 489-8787
  Herbs, herbals, herb and health books, juicers and small appliances.

Green Messenger Herbs
  P.O. Box U
  Hewitt, NJ 07421
  (201) 728-7835
  Excellent source of wildcrafted organic herbs, dry, tinctured, in formulas and salves. Books on herbs. Apprenticeships. Send SASE for catalogue.

For Lists of Doctors Using Nutritional Approaches to Health
The Life Extension Foundation
  (800) 841-LIFE

Resources for Information on Chronic Fatigue Immune Dysfunction Syndrome

Organizations:
CFIDS Activation Network
  P.O. Box 345
  Larchmont, NY 10538
  (212) 627-5631
  FAX (914) 636-6515
  CAN is an advocacy organization working to increase government research and aiming for effective treatment to correct the symptoms of CFIDS.

The CFIDS Association of America
P.O. Box 220398
Charlotte, NC 28222-0398
(800) 442-3437
(900) 896-2343
$2 for first minute, $1 for each additional minute. An information hotline including CFIDS monthly update and nutritional therapies. They have a journal, *The CFIDS Chronicle*, and are also a resource for books on CFIDS.

Books on CFIDS
CFIDS: The Disease with a Thousand Names
David Bell, M.D.
Pollard Publications, 1991
A comprehensive discussion with several chapters designed to aid doctors in treatment of CFIDS.

Hope and Help for Chronic Fatigue Syndrome
Karyn Feiden
Prentice Hall, 1992
Provides insight into the experience of having CFIDS and key strategies for treatment.

Running on Empty
Katrina Berne, Ph.D.
Hunter House Publishing, 1992
The author is a person with CFIDS and also a therapist. A good resource manual for physicians and sufferers of CFIDS.

Dr. Sherry Rogers
(800) 846-ONUS
For data and to order books by Dr. Sherry Rogers on E.I. and CFIDS.

Journal on CFIDS
Journal of the Chronic Fatigue Syndrome
  The Haworth Press
  Boc Comp
  10 Alice Street
  Binghamton, NY 13904
  Annual subscription, $28.

Computer Bulletin Board for People with CFIDS
  Send SASE to:

CFS Computer Network Project
  P.O. Box 2397
  Washington, DC 20008

RESOURCES FOR CHAPTER 5: EXERCISE

Books

The Complete Walker
Colin Fletcher
Knopf, 1992
The definitive book on hiking and backpacking with a good appendix listing hiking clubs and other resources.

Walking Medicine
Gary Yanker and Kathy Burton
McGraw-Hill, 1992
A walking program called Exercisewalking based on the advice of 35 medical experts.

Light on Yoga
B.K.S. Iyengar
Schocken, 1979
A classic. Very thorough description of the postures.

The Complete Illustrated Book of Yoga
  Swami Vishnu-devananda
  (800) 783-9642
  The bible of yogis. $14.95.

The Runner's Yoga Book
  Jean Couch
  Rodmell Press, 1991
  (510) 841-3123
  $18.95

Ancient Way to Keep Fit
  Compiled by Zong Wu
  Shelter Publications, 1992
  A guide to chi gung, an ancient Chinese exercise regime.

The Fitness Option: Five Weeks to Healing Stress
  Valerie O'Hara
  Dawn Publications, 1992
  A practical workbook to measure and overcome stress
  through exercise, breathing, yoga stretching.

Helping Yourself with Foot Reflexology
  Mildred Carter
  21st Century Publications
  (800) 593-2665

Tai Ji: Beginner's Tai Ji Book
  Al Huang Chungliang
  Celestial Arts, 1992
  An introductory book by a tai ji master to this Chinese
  exercise that is meditative and health-enhancing.

Living Yoga
  Edited by Georg Feuerstein and Stephan Bodian and the
  staff of *Yoga Journal*
  J.P. Tarcher, 1993

This is a collection of the most outstanding articles that have appeared in *Yoga Journal*; valuable both to newcomers and long-time practitioners.

Walking: The Complete Guide to the Complete Exercise
Casey Meyers
Random House, 1992
Tells how to maximize the benefits from the four basic walking speeds: stroll, brisk walk, aerobic walk, and race walking.

Kinesiology of Exercise
Michael Yessis
Masters Press, 1992
A guide to weight training suitable for all levels.

Stretching
Bob Anderson
Shelter Publications, 1980
A primer on stretching and limbering for the athlete at all fitness levels.

Magazines
Yoga Journal
2054 University Avenue
Berkeley, CA 94704
(415) 841-9200
$15 per year for 6 issues.

Walking
P.O. Box 52341
Boulder, CO 80321

Exercise Videos

The Sivananda Yoga Video
163 Amsterdam Avenue
New York, NY 10023
(800) 544-9852 ext. 492
For intermediate to advanced. $29.95.

Yoga Journal's Yoga
Healing Arts
321 Hampton Drive
Venice, CA 90291
(800) 722-7347
$59.98 for three 60-minute videos for intermediates.
$29.98 for Yoga for Beginners.

Iyengar on Video
Mystic River Video
P.O. Box 716
Cambridge, MA 02140
(617) 483-YOGA
Various two-tape sets featuring B.K.S. Iyengar—
Therapeutic Yoga, Teaching Teachers, and Questions and
Answers.

T'ai Chi for Health with Terry Dunn
Inerarts
279 South Beverly Drive
Beverly Hills, CA 90212
(800) 950-6002
$49.95 for two-hour video. Send $1 for catalogue.

Catalogues for Exercise Videos
Rudra Press
P.O. Box 1973
Cambridge, MA 02238
(800) 876-7798
Various video and audiotapes on tai chi and yoga.

Holistic Video Guide
The Holistic Arts and Sciences Network
P.O. Box 47855
Minneapolis, MN 55447

Wayfarer Publications
P.O. Box 26156
Los Angeles, CA 90026
(800) 888-9119
250 items related to tai chi, including Chinese martial arts videos, and books on philosophy and chi gung.

Equipment
Welles Enterprises
6565 Balboa Avenue, Suite A
San Diego, CA 92111
(800) 347-3881
The Welles Slant. A slant board, wood base with vinyl cover. Folds in half for storage. Lie on this for inversion beauty treatment or for exercise.

Inversion Swing
P.O. Box 2182
La Jolla, CA 92038
(800) 383-8056
Hang upside-down from this door-mounted inversion swing to hang out the back and reverse gravity. They have a catalogue.

BodyBridge
(800) 326-2724
Lying over this bridge with back arched backward releases tension and counters forward-bending hunch of writers and desk workers.

Yoga Schools

Jivamukti
149 Second Avenue
New York, NY 10003
(212) 353-0214
One of the best yoga schools anywhere.

Yoga Teachers Training Course
Sivananda Ashram Yoga Camp
Eighth Avenue
Val Morin, Quebec JOT 2RO
Canada
(819) 322-3226/(800) 783-9642
Ask about their yoga vacation and trainings in the Bahamas.

Walking Tours

Tre Laghi Travel (Swiss/Italian Walking Tour Specialists)
1536 N.W. 23rd Avenue
Portland, OR 97210
(800) 344-8890
Luxury walking tours.

Ryder-Walker Alpine Adventures
5 Lake Fork Junction
Box 947
Telluride, CO 81435
(303) 728-6481

Inn-to-inn trekking in the Swiss Alps or Scottish Highlands.

Backroads
1516 Fifth Street, Suite M7
Berkeley, CA 94710
(510) 527-1555/(800) 462-2848
Hiking tours.

Greenscape
Milkaway Lane
Croyde
North Devon EH33 ING
England
(011) 44 271 890677
(203) 322-1551 (Conn.)
Inn-to-inn walking tours of Cotswold Hills and the city of Bath led by a health practitioner, Dr. Morton Walker.

The Walker's Life
P.O. Box 16025
Lubbock, TX 79490
Information about peace walks.

Organization of Mall Walkers
P.O. Box 191
Hermann, MO 65041
Less romantic than the above, and certainly less full-spectrum light and oxygen, but still the benefits of walking. About 2,400 malls open early to accommodate walkers between 6:30 and 10 A.M.

Articles from Medical Journals on Exercise

"The Central and Peripheral Opoid Peptides"
N.H. Kalin
Psychiatric Clinics of North America: Symposium on Endorphins 6:421, Sept. 1983

"Endorphins and Exercise: A Review"
M.R. Forwood
The Australian Journal of Science and Medicine and Sports 63–65, Sept. 1991

"Exercise and the Heart"
C.J. Lavie
Postgraduate Medicine 91:130–48, Feb. 1, 1992

"Exercise, Fitness and Health: People Need to Be More Active More Often"
D. Cloag
British Medical Journal 305:377–78, Aug. 15, 1992

"Erythrocyte Free Radical Scavenger Enzymes in Professional Bicycle Racers"
P. Mena
International Journal of Sports Medicine 12:563–66, 1991

"Why Exercise?"
Per-Olaf Astrand
Medicine and Science and Sports and Exercise 24:153–62, 1992

"Antioxidant Reponse to Exercise: Induced Oxidative Stress and Protection of Vitamin E"
M. Meydani
Beyond Deficiency: New Views on the Function and Health Effects of Vitamins, New York Academy of Science, Feb. 9–12, 1992

"Women Walking for Health and Fitness: How Much Is Enough?"
Journal of American Medical Association 266:3295–99, Dec. 18, 1992

"Free Radicals, Antioxidants and Human Disease"
Barry Halliwell
Journal of Laboratory and Clinical Medicine 119:598–602, June 1992

RESOURCES FOR CHAPTER 6:
MIND OVER STRESS

Books
Getting Well Again
  Carl Simonton, M.D.
  Bantam Books, 1984
  Explains stress and mind-set as as contributing factors to
  the onset of disease, and gives techniques for relaxation.

The Healing Heart
  Norman Cousins
  Avon Books, 1983
  Tells how to utilize positive emotions and recounts his
  heart attack.

The Medium, the Mystic and the Physicist
Lawrence LeShan
Ballantine Books, 1974
Explains healing powers.

The Stress of Life
Hans Selye
McGraw-Hill, 1976
The first book on stress.

Healing and the Mind
Bill Moyers
Doubleday, 1993
The print companion to the PBS-TV series consists of 15 talks with researchers into mind-body healing methods. For the five videocassettes of the TV series call (800) 633-1999.

Mind-Body Medicine: How to Use Your Mind for Better Health
Daniel Goleman and Joel Gurin
Consumer Reports Books, 1992
This comprehensive 480-page book contains 25 chapters by leading experts in the field and is extremely useful.

Mind Matters: How the Mind and Brain Interact to Create Our Conscious Lives
Michael Gazzaniga
Houghton Mifflin, 1992

Psychoneuroimmunology
Robert Ader, David Felton, and Nicholas Cohen, editors
Academic Press, 1992
A compilation of research reports in the field of psychoneuroimmunology. This is the second edition; the first came out in 1981. $139.

Where the Mind Meets the Body
Harris Dienstfrey
HarperCollins, 1992

The Healing Brain
Robert Ornstein and David Sobel
Simon & Schuster, 1987
The authors believe the brain is "the key to health."

*Healing with Love: A Breakthrough Mind-Body Medical
Program for Healing Yourself and Others*
Leonard Laskow, M.D.
Harper & Row, 1986

The Healer Within
Steven Locke, M.D., and Douglas Colligan
Dutton, 1986

Creating Health
Deepak Chopra
Houghton Mifflin, 1987
He explains how "happy thoughts create health."

*Peace, Love and Healing: Body-Mind Communication and
the Path to Self-Healing: An Exploration*
Bernie Siegel, M.D.
Perennial Library, 1990

Head First: The Biology of Hope
Norman Cousins
Dutton, 1989
Establishes that emotions are biochemical reactions and
affirms the value of fostering healing attitudes.

Humor, Physiology and the Aging Process
William Fry
Humor and Aging, Academic Press, 1986, pp. 81–98
A synopsis of the physiology of humor.

*Change Your Mind, Change Your Life: Concepts in
Attitudinal Healing*
Gerald Jampolsky, M.D., and Diane Cirincione
Bantam Books, 1993
Points out that we can control our response, our attitudes
to life situations.

The Miracle of Mindfulness: A Manual on Meditation
Thich Nhat Hanh
Beacon Press, 1991
Hanh, a Vietnamese zen master and peace activist, gives
informal instructions on how to practice mindfulness.

A Guide to Walking Meditation
Thich Nhat Hanh
Fellowship of Reconciliation, 1985
The basics of walking meditation. Lovely book.

Journey of Awakening
Ram Dass
Bantam Books, 1978

How to Meditate
Larry LeShan
Bantam Books, 1975

A Gradual Awakening
Stephen Levine
Doubleday, 1979

*The Meditative Mind: The Varieties of Meditative
Experience*
Daniel Goleman
Tarcher, 1991
This book provides a description of the different types of
Eastern and Western meditation techniques.

The Pleasure Connection: How Endorphins Affect Our
Health and Happiness
Deva Beck and James Beck
Synthesis, 1992
This book clearly explains how endorphins function and
how we can stimulate them.

The Wisdom Within
Irving Oyle and Susan Jean
H.J. Kramer, 1993
This self-help book provides guidance on how to tap your
inner wisdom to access the benefits of mind-body
influence.

Spontaneous Remission: An Annotated Bibliography
Brendan O'Regan and Caryle Hirshberg
Institute of Noetic Sciences
This is the first survey to report on the phenomenon of
remission. It contains 1,574 references and covers the
entire spectrum of disease. $49 plus $4.25 postage.
Available from:
Institute of Noetic Sciences
P.O. Box 909
Sausalito CA 94966
(415) 331-5650/(800) 383-1586

Medical and Journal Articles

"Impact of a Dietary Change on Emotional Distress."
L. Christiansen et al.
Journal of Abnormal Pyschology 94:565–79, 1985

"Influence of Vitamin C Status on the Urinary Excretion of
Catecholamines in Stress"
A. Kallner
Human Nutrition 37:405–11, 1983

"Stress and Magnesium"
H. Classen
Artery 9:182–89, 1981

"The Concepts of Stress and Stress System Disorders"
G.P. Chrousos
Journal of the American Medical Association
267:1244–52, March 4, 1992

"Stress-Related Impairments in Cellular Immunity"
R. Glaser et al.
Psychiatry Research, 1985, pp. 233–39

"Stress Related Immune Suppression: Health Implications"
R. Glaser et al.
Brain, Behavior and Immunity, 1987, pp. 7–20

"Intangibles in Medicine: An Attempt at a Balancing
Perspective"
Journal of the American Medical Association, 1988, pp.
1610–12

"Psychoneuroimmunology: Toward a Mind-Body Model"
Kenneth Pelletier and Denise Herzing
Advances, 1988, pp. 27–56

"Psychoneuroimmunology: Interactions Between Central
Nervous System and Immune System"
Journal of Neuroscience Research, 1987, pp. 1–9

"The Concepts of Stress and Stress System Disorders:
Overview of Physical and Behavioral Homeostasis"
George Chrousos and Philip Gold
Journal of American Medical Association, March 4,
1992, pp. 1244–52

"Lymphocyte Production of Endorphins and Endorphin Mediated Immunoregulatory Activity"
Eric Smith et al.
American Association of Immunologists, 1985, pp. 770–82

"Peptide Hormones Shared by the Neuroendocrine and Immunologic Systems"
Edwin Blalock et al.
American Association of Immunologists, 1985, pp. 858–61

"Psychoneuroendocrine Influences on Immunocompetence and Neoplasia"
Riley Vernon
Science, June 1981, p. 1100

"Strong Emotional Response to Disease May Bolster Patients' Immune System"
New York Times, Oct. 22, 1985, p. C1

"Sense of Humor as a Moderator of the Relation Between Stressors and Moods"
Dr. Road Martin and Herbert Lefcourt
Journal of Personality and Social Psychology, 1983, pp. 1313–24

"Personal Health: Increasingly, Laughter as Potential Therapy for Patients Is Being Taken Seriously"
Jane Brody
New York Times, April 7, 1988

"Neuropeptides and Their Receptors: A Psychosomatic Network"
C.B. Pert et al.
Journal of Immunology, 1985

"Neuropeptides: The Emotions and Beyond"
C.B. Pert
Noetic Sciences Review, Spring 1987

Immune System Changes During Humor Associated Laughter
L.S. Berk
Dept. of Pathology and Laboratory Medicine, 1990

Meditation Tapes
Mind-Body Health Sciences
393 Dixon Road
Selma Star Rte.
Boulder, CO 80302
(303) 440-8460
Guided meditation tapes from Joan Borysenko.

If the following tapes on meditation are not in your local store, they are available from:

Yes! Books and Video
P.O. Box 10726
Arlington, VA 2210
(800) YES-0234

How to Meditate
Lawrence LeShan, Ph.D.
A one-hour tape that guides you through four meditations with a 32-page guide.

Five Classic Meditations
Shinzen Young
A variety of meditations from several traditions.

The Meditative Mind
Daniel Goleman
A one-hour tape leads you through four meditations.

Alpha Meditation—Focal Point
Modern sound technology with special tones helps to put
you into a meditative alpha state.

The Practice of Mindfulness in Psychotherapy
Thich Nhat Hanh
This three-hour tape set focuses on how to work with
anger through breathing and walking meditation.

Inner Vision: Visualizing Super Health
with Bernie Siegel, Gerald Kamplosky, and Norman
Shealy
This 40-minute video illustrates the practice and use of
various visualization techniques, and contains an extended
visualization. $49.95 plus postage.

Quantum Healing: Toward Perfect Healing
Deepak Chopra
This 35-minute videotape includes discussion of pioneers
in holistic health and current findings in mind-body
research. $30 plus postage.

Both *Inner Vision* and *Quantum Healing* available from:
Institute of Noetic Sciences
P.O. Box 909
Sausalito CA 94966-0909
(415) 331-5650/(800) 383-1586

Journals on Mind-Body and Stress

Advances: The Journal of Mind-Body Health
9292 West KL Avenue
Kalamazoo, MI 49009
(616) 375-2000
A scholarly journal examining mind's influence on the body. Quarterly, $39.

Brain, Behavior and Immunity
Academic Press
1250 Sixth Avenue
San Diego, CA 92101-9923
(619) 230-1840
Quarterly, $160.

Noetic Sciences Review
Institute of Noetic Sciences
P.O. Box 909, Dept. M
Sausalito, CA 94966-0909
(800) 383-1394
Discusses new concepts in mind and consciousness research. Quarterly. Membership includes the journal. $35.

Catalogues of Books and Audio- and Videotapes Related to Mind-Body, Stress and Healing, Meditation, and More

Yes! Books and Video
P.O. Box 10726
Arlington, VA 22210
(800) YES-0234

Samuel Weiser, Inc.
132 East 24th Street
New York, NY 10010
(212) 777-6363

The Sounds True Catalog
735 Walnut Street
Dept. FC5
Boulder, CO 80302
(800) 333-9185

An Intelligent Guide
Institute of Noetic Sciences
P.O. Box 909
Sausalito, CA 94966-0909
(800) 383-1394
Their excellent catalogue comes with membership,
$35.00; in addition you will get their bulletin, *Noetic
Sciences*.

Pacific Spirit
1334 Pacific Avenue
Forest Grove, OR 97116
(800) 634-9057

Mystic Fire Video
P.O. Box 2249
Livonia, MI 48151
(800) 292-9001
A catalogue of illuminating videos on consciousness,
healing, art, and myth.

Parallax Press
P.O. Box 7355
Berkeley, CA 94707
(510) 525-0101
Books and videos on the practice of mindfulness.

Humoresource: A Collection of Jest-Sellers on Humor
110 Spring Street
Saratoga Springs, NY 12866
(518) 587-8770
Over 200 books, audiotapes, videos, computer software
that will cultivate a laugh and good humor. How to
utilize humor in business and creativity.

Newsletters

Brain/Mind Bulletin
P.O. Box 42211
Los Angeles, CA 90042
(213) 223-2500/(800) 553-MIND
$45 for a subscription, 12 issues. They also have
collections of their articles by topic—for instance mind
and immunity, personal energy, and athletics—for prices
ranging from $20 to $30.

The Mindfulness Bell
Community of Mindful Living
Parallax Press
P.O. Box 7355
Berkeley, CA 94707
(510) 525-0101
Newsletter for the community of mindful living. Each
monthly issue contains a talk by Thich Nhat Hanh, a
Buddhist monk, and listenings of local practice groups
and retreat schedules. $12.

Learn to Utilize the Alpha State
Silva Mind Method
P.O. Box 187
Murray Hill Station
New York, NY 10156-0187
(212) 490-2400
OR

Silva International
1407 Calle del Norte
P.O. Box 2249
Laredo, TX 78044-2249
(210) 722-6391
The four-day Silva course teaches you to enter the relaxed-mind-functioning state called alpha and to utilize its intuitive and creative capacity to manage stress and enhance your life and health. Success stories of the graduates are inspiring.

The Healing Power of Music

The following tapes and CDs help to remove the blocks to healing and they invigorate the spirit. They are available from:
Sounds True Catalogue
735 Walnut Street
Boulder, CO 80302
(303) 449-6229

Healing Music from China
Gregorian Chants, by the Deller Consort
The Songs the Plants Taught Us: Authentic Healing Music from Peru
Sacred Healing Chants from Tibet: The Monks of the Gaden Shartse Monastery

Books on Aromatherapy

The Complete Book of Essential Oils and Aromatherapy
Valerie Ann Worwood
New World Library, 1991
California

Aromatherapy. An A to Z
C.W. Daniel, 1988
England

The Aromatherapy Workbook
Marcel Lavabre
Healing Arts Press, 1990
Vermont

RESOURCES FOR CHAPTER 7: LIGHT

Books on Light
Color Healing—Chromotherapy
  By leading authors in the field
  Contains a condensation of the famous book *The Principles of Light and Color* by Edwin Babbit.

The Seven Keys to Color Healing
  Roland Hunt

The above two books are available from:
21st Century Publications
P.O. Box 702
Fairfield, IA 52556
(515) 472-5105/(800) 593-2665

Rise of the Phoenix
Dr. Christopher Hills
Common Ownership Press, 1979, p. 1012
Boulder, CO

Health and Light
John Ott
Pocket Books, 1976

Light, Radiation and You
John Ott
P.O. Box 40004
Crescent Beach
Sarasota, FL 34242
Enclose SASE.

Nuclear Evolution
Dr. Christopher Hills
University of the Trees Press, 1977
Boulder, CO

The Secret of Light
Walter Russell
University of Science and Philosophy, 1974
Charlottesville, VA 22901

Colour
Rudolf Steiner
Rudolf Steiner Press, 1982
London

The Medical and Biological Effects of Light
Richard Wurtman
The New York Academy of Sciences, 1985

Biological Effects of Ultraviolet Radiation
Walter Harm
Cambridge University Press, 1980

Sunlight
Zane Kime, M.D.
World Health Publications, 1980

Light: Medicine of the Future
Jacob Liberman
Bear and Company, 1991

Day Light Robbery
Dr. Damien Downing
Arrow Books, 1988

Sunlight and Health
Michael Lillyquist
Dodd, Mead, 1985

Articles on Light
"The Effects of Color on Human Behavior"
J.J. Plank
Journal of Association for Study of Perception, 1974, pp. 4–16

"Melatonin Extends Rat Lives"
W. Pierpaoli
Brain/Mind Bulletin, June 1988, pp. 1–8

"The Pineal Gland: An Important Link to the Environment"
R.J. Reiter
NIPS, Dec. 1986, pp. 202–5

"Effect of Ultraviolet Light on Physical Fitness"
R.M. Allen
Archives of Physical Medicine, 1945, pp. 641–44

"Effects of Spectral Differences in Illumination on Fatigue"
J.B. Mass
Journal of Applied Psychology, 1974, pp. 524–26

"The Effects of Light on the Human Body"
R.J. Wurtmann
Scientific American, 1975

"Immunological Effects of Solarium Exposure"
Peter Hersey
Lancet, March 12, 1983, pp. 545–48

"Cumulative Effects of Repeated Subthreshold Doses of
Ultraviolet Radiation"
John Parrish
Journal of Investigative Dermatology, 1981, pp. 356–58

"Malignant Melanoma and Exposure to Fluorescent
Lighting at Work"
Valerie Beral
Lancet, Aug. 7, 1982, pp. 290–93

"Effects of Wavelengths of Light on Physiological
Functions of Plants and Animals"
John Ott
Illuminating Eng, 1965, pp. 254–61

"Color and Light: Their Effects on Plants, Animals, and
People"
John Ott
International Journal of Biosocial Research, 10, 1988,
pp. 111–116, 126, 127

"School Lights and Problem Pupils"
Joan Arehart-Treichel
Science News, April 20, 1974

"Surprising Health Impact Discovered for Light"
Jane Brody
New York Times, Nov. 13, 1984

"Shedding Light on Dark-Day Blues"
Georgia Dullea
New York Times, Dec. 29, 1985

"Exposure to Sun Helps Prevent Cancer Deaths"
Science Newsletter, 1940, pp. 198–99

"Seasonal Affective Disorder: A Description of the
Syndrome and Preliminary Findings with Light Therapy"
N.E. Rosenthal
Archives of General Psychiatry, 1984, pp. 72–80

"Influence of Graduated Sunlight Baths on Patients with
Coronary Atherosclerosis"
V.A. Mikhailov
Soviet Medicine, 1966, p. 76

Resources for Lighting
The Sun Box Company
  1100 Tfat Street
  Rockville, MD 20850
  (800) 548-3968
  FAX (301) 762-8956
  In addition to publishing the *SunNet News*, a quarterly
  newsletter on light they sell various light fixtures
  including a light visor (to be worn on the head just 30
  minutes a day), a sunbox ($399), screw-in fluorescent
  full-spectrum bulbs, a sunlight pipe to be fit into the
  ceiling to bring in outdoor light ($399), and other items.

NEEDS (National Ecological and Environmental Delivery System)
527 Charles Avenue, 12A
Syracuse, NY 13209
(800) 634-1380
For Chromolux bulbs and other excellent health-related products. Get their catalogue.

Medic Light
Yacht Club Drive
Lake Hopatcong, NJ 07849
(201) 663-1214
They make a light box system in various sizes for desk or floor.

Befit Enterprises
Southampton, NY 11969
(516) 287-3813
(800) 497-9516
They sell Chromalux color corrected bulbs, the OTT-Lite fixture, and other environmental stress reduction equipment. Get their catalogue.

OTT-Lite Systems
306 East Cota Street
Santa Barbara, CA 93101
(800) 234-3724
Ask for the OTT-Lite.

Duro-Test
9 Law Drive
Fairfield, NJ 07007
(800) 289-3876
Ask for Vita-Lite (full-spectrum fluorescent).

Sunsor UV System
  Sunsor, Inc.
  1388 Freeport Road
  Pittsburgh, PA 15238
  (412) 967-0580
  A small hand-held meter to measure UVB and an
  exposure guide for five basic types of skin sensitivity. In
  the $30 range. Contact above for retail outlet.

Suggestions for SAD (Seasonal Affective Disorder)
Society for Light Treatment
  P.O. Box 478
  Wilsonville, OR 97070
  (503) 694-2404
  Quarterly bulletin of the society is $15; SAD Information
  Packet is $7 (includes bibliography and a list of research
  centers and clinicians); membership in the society is $60
  (regular), $10 (student).

Professional Publications on SAD
Seasonal Affective Disorders and Phototherapy
  N. Rosenthal and M. Blehar
  Guilford Press, NY, 1989

Seasonal Affective Disorder
  C. Thompson and T. Silverstone
  Sheridan Medical Book Publishers
  145 Palisades Street
  Dobbs Ferry, NY 10522
  Or Clinical Neuroscience Publishers, London, 1989

"Phototherapy for Season Affective Disorders in Alaska"
  C.J. Hellekson, M.D.
  University of Alaska American Journal of Psychiatry 143:
  1035–37, August 1986

"Bright Artificial Light Treatment of a Manic Depressive
Patient with Seasonal Mood Cycle"
A.J. Lewy
American Journal of Psychiatry 139:1496–98, 1982

Books on SAD
*SAD: Winter Depression: Who Gets It, What Causes It, and
How to Cure It*
A. Smyth
HarperCollins, 1991

*Seasons of the Mind: Why You Get Winter Blues and What
You Can Do About It*
N.E. Rosenthal
Bantam Books, 1989

Resource on Ozone
Ozone Action
  34 Wall Street, Suite 203
  Asheville, NC 28801
  (704) 254-3811
  Ozone Action is dedicated to educating the public about
  the human and environmental harm caused by UV
  radiation, with a view toward halting the destruction of
  the ozone layer.

RESOURCES FOR CHAPTER 8: POLLUTION

Organizations
Americans for Safe Food
  1501 16th Street, N.W.
  Washington, DC 20036
  For booklets listing mail-order organic food, and guidance
  on how to petition your grocery to carry organic foods.

National Coalition Against the Misuse of Pesticides
  530 7th Street, S.E.
  Washington, DC 20003
  (202) 543-5450
  A national network committed to encouraging alternative
  pest management.

Organic Foods Production Association
125 West 7th Street
Wind Gap, PA 18091
(215) 863-6700
For information on organic foods.

Public Citizen
215 Pennsylvania Avenue, S.E.
Washington, DC 20003
(202) 546-4996
A nonprofit citizens group concerned with food safety and other crucial issues. Join up, get their literature.

Information on Pesticides in Foods and Guides to Actions

Rachel Carson Council
8940 Jones Mill Road
Chevy Chase, MD 20815
(301) 652-1877
International resource center on pesticide information.

California Action Network
P.O. Box 464
Davis, CA 95617
(916) 756-8518
Organic Wholesalers Directory and Yearbook. Lists resources for organic foods. $19 plus $1.75 s&h.

National Pesticide Telecommunication Network
(800) 858-PEST/(800) 858-7378

EPA Emergency Planning and Community Right-to-Know Hotline
(800) 535-0202
They will provide information on hazardous chemicals used by local businesses.

National Pesticide Telecommunications Network
  Texas University Health Science Center
  School of Medicine
  Lubbock, TX 79430
  (800) 858-PEST
  A pesticide hotline for product symptoms, toxicity,
  safety, health effects, and other information.

National Resources Defense Council
  40 West 20th Street
  New York, NY 10114
  (212) 727-2700
  Reports on food hazards and pesticides.

Books on Pollution

Safe Food: Eating Wisely in a Risky World
  Michael Jacobson, Lisa Lefferts, and Anne Witte Garland
  Center Science Public Interest and Living Planet Press,
  1991

The Artist's Complete Health and Safety Guide
  Monona Rossol
  Allsworth Press, NY, 1990

Silent Spring
  Rachel Carson
  Houghton Mifflin, 1962
  Anniversary Edition, 1987

The Recurring Silent Spring
  Patricia Hayes
  Pergamon Press, 1989

*Defusing the Toxic Threat: Controlling Pesticides and
Industrial Waste*
Sandra Postel
Worldwatch Institute, Dec. 1988
1776 Massachusetts Avenue
Washington, DC 20036
69 pages, $4.

*Empty Harvest: Understanding the Link Between Our Food,
Our Immunity and Our Planet*
Dr. Bernard Jensen and Mark Anderson
Avery Publishing Group, 1991
(800) 548-5757

The Pesticide Conspiracy
Robert van den Bosch
Anchor Books, 1978
Out of print but may be found in libraries.

Herbal Mosquito Repellents
Lakon Herbals
Box 252
Montpelier, VT 05601
Sells Bygone Bugs.

Green Ban
Box 146
Norway, IA 52318

Testing for Environmental Problems
R.C.I. Environmental
Dallas, TX
(214) 250-6609 (Marti)
They have kits for testing water, indoor air quality,
pesticides, formaldehyde, asbestos, mold. Also help with
power line transformers leaking, etc.

Environmental Outfitters
44 Crosby Street
New York, NY 10012
(800) 238-5008
They provide clean, safe building materials, including paints and flooring and also state-of-the-art water and air filtration. They have consulting services to test your home.

EPA Hazardous Waste Hotline
(800) 424-9346
Call them for information.

Resources for Mercury Toxicity
Dr. Victor Penzer
197 Grant Avenue
Newton Center, MA 02159
(617) 332-1324

Coalition of Mercury Amalgam Victims
P.O. Box 458
Allston, MA 02134
(617) 536-4966

Toxic Testing
303 East Altamonte Drive, Suite 232
Altamonte Springs, FL 32701
(800) 327-8885
List of mercury-free dentistry practitioners.

Books on Mercury Toxicity
A Patient's Guide to Mercury Amalgam Toxicity
Roy Kupsinel
self-published

available from:
P.O. Box 550
Oviedo, FL 32767
(305) 365-6681

*The Toxic Time Bomb: Can the Mercury in Your Dental
Fillings Poison You?*
Sam Ziff
Aurora Press
Box 573
Santa Fe, NM 87504
(505) 989-9804

Books on Nuclear Issues

Deadly Deceit: Low-Level Radiation, High-Level Cover-up
Dr. Jay Gould and Benjamin Goldman
Four Walls Eight Windows, NY 1990
(800) 444-2524
Must reading!

The Petkau Effect
Dr. Graueb
Four Walls Eight Windows, 1992
(800) 444-2524
Must reading!

*Mother Country: Britain, the Welfare State and Nuclear
Pollution*
Marilynne Robinson
Farrar, Straus and Giroux, 1989
A brilliant work of investigative reporting on the
Sellafield Reprocessing Plant in England, which
discharges 15 million gallons of radioactive water daily
into the Irish Sea.

*Nuclear Legacy: Overview of Plants, Problems and Politics
of Radioactive Waste in the United States*
Scott Saleska
Published by Public Citizen, 1989
215 Pennsylvania Avenue, S.E.
Washington, DC 20003
$23.

Radiation Induced Cancer from Low Dose Exposure
John Gofman, M.D., Ph.D.
Available from:
The Committee for Nuclear Responsibility
P.O. Box 11207
San Francisco, CA 94101
Written by the professor emeritus of medical physics at
Berkeley, this book provides irrefutable proof that,
contrary to industry claims, even the lowest possible
doses of ionizing radiation are carcinogenic. It discusses
the practice of altering data retroactively after results are
known, suppressing the unaltered data, and the conflict of
interest in health research.
$29.95 plus $4 postage.

No Immediate Danger
Rosalie Bertell, Ph.D.
Available from:
International Institute of Concern for Public Health
630 Bathurst Street
Toronto, Ontario M5R 3GI
Canada
A stunning, honest evaluation of nuclear history, and an
inspiring call to action. $17.95 plus s&h. *Highly
recommended!*

*Macrocosm USA: An Environmental, Political and Social
Solutions Handbook with Directories*
Foreword by Marilyn Ferguson
Edited by Sandi Brockway
Available from:
Macrocosm USA
P.O. Box 969
Cambria, CA 93428
A good resource book for people, organizations,
computers, media, periodicals, and more. Includes essays
on environment-related topics.

Diet for the Atomic Age
Sara Shannon
Avery Publishing Group, 1987
(800) 548-5757
A clear history of the nuclear industry, radiation health
damage, and how to utilize "radio-protective" foods.
Unique 30 pages of medical and scientific references.

*Cover-up: What You Are Not Supposed to Know About
Nuclear Power*
Karl Grossman
Permanent Press, Sag Harbor, NY, 1982
Excellent book.

Plutonium
Stanley Berne and Arlene Zekowski
Order from:
Rising Tide Press
P.O. Box 6136
Santa Fe, NM 87502
(800) 247-6553
This book, focusing on plutonium, covers every facet of
the industry. $10.95 plus $2.50 s&h.

Radiation and Chernobyl: This Generation and Beyond
John Gofman, M.D., Ph.D.
Committee for Nuclear Responsibility, 1994
To order:
Committee for Nuclear Responsibility
P.O. Box 4 1993
San Francisco, CA 94142

American Ground Zero (The Secret Nuclear War)
Carole Gallagher
The MIT Press, 1993
To order, send $53 to:
The MIT Press/Order Dept.
55 Hayward Street
Cambridge, MA 02142
(800) 356-0343
A book of photographs and interviews with people who
were exposed to the fallout from the atmospheric bomb
testing in Nevada during the 1950s.

Films and Videos

The sources listed below have a variety of films and videos
relating to nuclear power, weapons, and health.

Direct Cinema
P.O. Box 315
Franklin Lakes, NJ 07417
(201) 891-8240
Catalogue available on request.

EnviroVideo
Box 311
Ft. Tilden, NY 11695
(718) 318-7715

EnviroVideo features documentaries on the nuclear industry, renewable energies, the nuclearization of space, and chemical-free farming. Suggested: *Three Mile Island Revisited*, which utilizes testimony of area residents and scientific findings to reveal that deaths, especially from cancer, and birth defects in children have been widespread since the 1979 accident at the Pennsylvania nuclear facility. VHS copies, $14.75 plus $2.25 s&h. Also available on ¾-inch videotape suitable for cable TV for $30.

Green Mountain Post Films
P.O. Box 229
Turner's Falls, MA 01376
(413) 863-4754/(413) 863-8248
Catalogue available on request.

Parallel Films
314 West 91st Street
New York, NY 10024
(212) 580-3888
Brochures and further information available on request.

Computerized Databases
NARMIC (National Action/Research on the Military Industrial Complex)
A Project of the American Friends Service Committee
1501 Cherry Street
Philadelphia, PA 19102
(215) 241-7175
A research and resource publication division of the American Friends Service Committee, NARMIC provides detailed information about Pentagon contracting and companies doing military work.

Nuclear Information and Resource Service
1616 P Street, N.W., Suite 160
Washington, DC 20036
(202) 328-0002
The computerized bulletin board NIRSNET provides daily updates on news regarding legislation, the Nuclear Regulatory Commission, and issues of relevance to antinuclear activists.

Nuclear Operations Analysis Center
P.O. Box Y
Oak Ridge National Laboratory
Oak Ridge, TN 37831
(615) 574-0391
Funded primarily by the NRC, this computer service provides information on reactor safety and operations.

PeaceNet
1918 Bonita
Berkeley, CA 94704
(415) 486-0264
A global computer-based communications and information-sharing system designed to increase the effectiveness of the peace, environmental, and social justice movements, PeaceNet enables individuals and organizations to gain access to and post information about antinuclear projects and events.

Periodicals

Downtown
151 First Avenue
New York, NY 10003
(212) 529-2255
This biweekly newspaper is *must* reading for the latest enviro-information. Read the "Eco-Frontier" column by

Harold Egeln for the most current news in the country on topics not discussed but touching us all in relation to the demise of Mother Earth. They are a national paper so perhaps you can request distribution in your area, or get a subscription.

War and Peace Digest
32 Union Square East
New York, NY 10003
A bimonthly newsletter on environmental and related issues. Up-to-date coverage. One-year subscription, $18.

Committee for Nuclear Responsibility
P.O. Box 421993
San Francisco, CA 94142
Gifts for the committee's work are tax-deductible and will also provide you with a newsletter of important information. Suggested donations of $25 or $50.

Natural Rights
The Natural Rights Center
P.O. Box 90
Summertown, TX 38483
An excellent quarterly newsletter with facts about our habitat, $30.

Monitors for Low-Level Radiation
Call to get information and catalogue from the following:

International Medcom
7497 Kennedy Road
Sebastopol, CA 95472
(707) 823-0336
The RadAlert is a handy, dependable, hand-sized low-level radiation monitor. About $290 plus s&h. They also

have a low-cost probe for environment education, $79.
Recently developed is the Vista 1600 probe for outdoor
use, which monitors the gasses emitted from nuclear
plants. It is hooked up to a computer and continuously
records radiation levels. Cost is from $1,000 up.
Greenpeace and many environmental groups use their
instruments.

Dosimeter Corporation
1286 Brooms Road
Cincinnati, OH 45242
(513) 489-8100
They have monitors in various sizes and prices.

Monitors and Detectors
26930 State Route 1
Guilford, IN 47022
(800) 637-2126
Dosimeters for personal monitoring, $110 to $200.

SE International
P.O. Box 39
436 Farm Road
Summertown, TN 38483
(615) 964-3561
They have seven different types of lightweight personal
monitors, $226 to $400.

Citizen Monitoring of Nuclear Power Plant Releases
Citizen Monitoring Network
115 High Street
Bath, ME 04530
(207) 443-3588
Call to get advice on how to set up a monitoring system
in your area to keep track of releases from nuclear plants.

There are a few groups around the country doing this. TMI set up an excellent system in 1993 using the International Medcom instruments (see above for address).

Organizations Working for Safe Energy
The following have excellent booklets and newsletters. Join up!

Greenpeace Action
  1436 U Street, N.W., Suite 201-A
  Washington, DC 20009
  (201) 462-8817

Nuclear Information and Resource Service (NIRS)
  1424 16th Street, N.W., Suite 601
  Washington, DC 20036
  (202) 328-0002

Safe Energy Communication Council (SECC)
  1717 Massachusetts Avenue, N.W., Suite LL215
  Washington, DC 20036
  (202) 483-8491

Public Citizen Critical Mass Energy Project
  215 Pennsylvania Avenue, S.E.
  Washington, DC 20003
  (202) 546-4996

Eco News Services
EcoNet
  3228 Sacramento Street
  San Francisco, CA 94115
  (415) 442-0220
  Computer information service.

Environmental News Service
3505 West 15th Avenue
Vancouver, BC V6R 2Z3
Canada
(604) 732-4000

News Travel Network
747 Front Street
San Francisco, CA 94111
(415) 397-2876
IMPACT Environmental reports. Provides on-location
enviro-reports for TV.

Environmental Software
Chariot Software Group
3659 India Street
San Diego, CA 92103
(619) 298-0202
Contact them for various educational environmental
software.

Alternate Energy
International Tesla Society
P.O. Box 5636
Colorado Springs, CO 809311
(719) 475-0918
Leaders in the field of alternate energy, they have a
catalogue of books and information on alternative energy
and environmentally friendly systems. Send $5 for a
sample of their magazine, *Extraordinary Science*, and a
packet of information. They are represented in 22
countries.

International Association for New Science
  1304 South College Avenue
  Fort Collins, CO 80524
  (303) 482-3731
  Their purpose is to promote a new science that will help
  the evolvement of mankind and initiate a paradigm shift.
  Membership ($30) includes the quarterly *New Science*
  news and information regarding conferences.

Tesla Said
  Compiled by John Ratzlaff
  Tesla Book Company, 1992
  This is a collection of articles and papers of Nikola Tesla,
  the early twentieth-century leader in the electrical field.
  It is available from:
  Tesla Book Co.
  PO Box 121873
  Chula Vista, CA 91912
  (800) 398-2056
  Also ask for their list of books.

Sunelco Solar
  P.O. Box 1499
  Hamilton, MO 59840-1499
  (800) 338-6844
  They distribute photovoltaic modules, inverters,
  controllers, and water pumps, and they design
  independent home energy systems.

Solar Energy Industries Association
  777 Number Capitol Street
  Washington, DC 20002
  A trade group for solar energy. Get their directory, *Solar
  Source Book*, $12.50.

Sun-Mate Corporation
  8110 Remmet Avenue
  Canoga Park, CA 91304
  (818) 883-7766
  They sell solar-powered consumer products.

Rocky Mountain Institute
  1739 Snowmass Creek Road
  Snowmass, CO 81654
  (303) 927-3128
  Key resource for research and information on alternate
  energy and how to live "off the grid."

Real Goods
  966 Mazzoni Street
  Ukiah, CA 95482-3471
  (800) 762-7325
  They produce an excellent catalogue on materials and
  products for alternate energy and energy conservation,
  The Real Goods Catalog. Their 60-page quarterly
  newsletter, *The Real Goods News*, is full of leads for
  efficient living and sensible energy use. Also look into
  their *Alternate Energy Sourcebook*.

*The Independent Home—Living Well with Power from the
  Sun, Wind and Water*
  Michael Potts
  Real Goods Trading, 1993
  This book features homes and people who are living off
  the grid. They rely on power from the sun, wind and
  water, using renewable technologies to reverse power
  dependancy. The book contains 60 photos of these homes
  and 35 illustrations that demonstrate the technologies.
  Inspiring!

Available from:
Real Goods
966 Mazzoni Street
Ukiah CA 95482
($18 plus postage)
(800) 762-7325

Background Reading
Energy and War
L.H. and A.B. Lovins
Friends of the Earth, 1980

Radon Tests
There are two main types of radon detectors: charcoal canister and alpha track detector. Measurements will be reported either in working levels (WL) or picocuries per liter (pCi/L).

Two companies that have been validated by the EPA:

Radon Testing Corporation of America
P.O. Box 258
Irvington, NY 10533
(800) 457-2366
They do residential and commercial testing for radon.
They send you a canister, which you place in your home and then return to them for analysis.

Teledyne Isotopes
50 Van Buren Avenue
Westwood, NJ 07675
(800) 666-0222
They do radon testing. They send a canister with full instructions. You place the canister in your home for four days, then return to them for analysis. $30 for one canister.

Sources for professional help on high radon levels:

Environmental Outfitters
  44 Crosby Street
  New York, NY 10012
  (800) 238-5008
  They have consulting services to test your home. They also design and sell building materials that are nontoxic.

Radon Information Hotline
  (800) 767-7326

Ozone
Ozone Action
  34 Wall Street, Suite 203
  Asheville, NC 28801
  (704) 254-3811
  Ozone Action is dedicated to informing the public about the human and environmental harm caused by UV radiation, with a view toward halting the destruction of the ozone layer.

Organizations Concerned with Food Irradiation
Food and Water, Inc.
  Old Schoolhouse Common
  R.D. 1, Box 30
  Marshfield, VT 05658
  (802) 426-3700/(800) EAT-SAFE
  A consumer advocacy organization focusing on safe food and water. They have been especially concerned about food irradiation and are active in disseminating information to the public. Subscribe to their newsletter, *Safe Food News*.

Health and Energy Institute
236 Massachusetts Avenue, Suite 506
Washington, DC 20002
(202) 543-1070

The Coalition to Stop Food Irradiation
P.O. Box 590488
San Francisco, CA 94159

Center for Food Safety and Applied Nutrition
Food and Drug Administration
200 C Street, N.W.
Washington, DC 20204
(202) 205-4850
Comments on food irradiation can be directed to the
FDA.

For ELF Radiation Monitoring
Spectrum Pro-Health
61 Dutile Road
Laconia, NH 03246
(603) 528-4710
Their BioSafe meter measures magnetic, electrical, and
microwave radiation, $145.95. Their AlphaLab magnetic
scanner measures magnetic radiation, $49.95.

Health Star
1800 South Robertson Boulevard
Los Angeles, CA 90035
(213) 838-5675
The Power Pet. This device reads green for safe and red
for warning, $39.95.

Teslatronics
One Progress Boulevard, Suite 25
Alachua, FL 32615
(904) 462-2010
Various ELF meters from $119 to $450.

Tools for Exploration
4286 Redwood Highway, Suite CY
San Rafael, CA 94903
(415) 499-9050
Measures electric fields, magnetic fields, and radio and microwaves in all directions simultaneously. $99.50 plus $5.50 s&h.

Publications on ELF
VDT News
Microwave News
P.O. Box 1799, Grand Central Station
New York, NY 10163
(212) 517-2802

EMF Bioeffects Database Information Ventures
1500 Locust Street, Suite 3216
Philadelphia, PA 19102
(215) 732-9083

Companies That Test for EMF
Safe Environments
2512 9th Street
Berkeley, CA 94710
(415) 549-9693

National EMF Testing Association
  628-B Liberty Place
  Evanston, IL 60201
  (708) 475-3696

EMF Measuring Services
  Manchester, MA
  (508) 526-4192

Environmental Electrics
  1618 Grand Avenue
  San Rafael, CA 94901
  (415) 454-8408

Devices to Neutralize ELF

ELF damage is due to random chaotic energy. There are systems engineered to organize these disordered fields in a certain area. They do not lower the levels, but they do organize the random photons.

Borderland Sciences Research Foundation
  P.O. Box 429
  Garberville, CA 95542
  Their Spacecrafter device is intended to clear
  electromagnetic fields that disturb living things and
  eliminate biological stress, $500.

Clarus Systems
  3901 MacArthur Boulevard, Suite 200
  Newport Beach, CA 92660
  They have systems for home, car, workplace, computer,
  and video. Clarus Environment System. VDT clear (for
  VDT monitor). CarClear (for car interior). Video Clear
  (for TV/VCR video systems).

The Energy Group
  346 Oakhurst Drive
  Beverly Hills, CA 90210
  (310) 859-8895
  A clock that plugs in and clears electric currents.

Ener-G Polari-T Products
  P.O. Box 2449
  Prescott, AZ 86302
  (602) 778-5039
  They make products that maintain the body's electrical
  balance. Free catalogue.

VDT (Video Display Terminal) Protection
I-Protect Inc.
  6151 West Century Boulevard, Suite 916
  Los Angeles, CA 90045
  (213) 215-1664
  A shield that blocks radiation and UV that may be
  emitted from the monitor's cathode ray.

Safe Computing Company
  368 Hillside Avenue
  Needham, MA 02194
  (800) 222-3003

Safe Technologies Corporation
  1950 N.E. 208 Terrace
  North Miami Beach, FL 33179
  (800) 639-9121
  Safe computer monitors.

Books and Articles on EMF
Cross Currents
  Robert Becker
  Tarcher, 1990

"Annals of Radiation: The Hazards of EMF's"
Paul Brodeur
The New Yorker, June 12, 1989, pp. 51–88, and June 19, pp. 47–73

Currents of Death
Paul Brodeur
Simon and Schuster, 1989

The Great Power Line Cover-Up
Paul Brodeur
Little, Brown and Company, 1993

EPA Draft Review: Evaluation of the Potential Carcinogenicity of Electromagnetic Fields
Office of Research and Development
Washington, DC, October 1990

Case Control Study of Childhood Cancer and Residential Exposure to Electric and Magnetic Fields
David Savitz
Final report to the New York Power Lines Project, 1986

"Electrical Wiring Configurations and Childhood Cancer"
Nancy Wertheimer
American Journal of Epidemiology 109, pp. 273–84, 1979

Warning: The Electricity Around You May Be Hazardous
Ellen Sugarman
Simon & Schuster, 1992

Citizen Groups
Electromagnetic Pollution Society (EMPAS)
P.O. Box 60
Burns Lake, BC VOJ, 1EO
Canada
(604) 694-3740

Citizens Concerned About EMF's
P.O. Box 120
San Ramon, CA 94583

Citizens Against Overhead Power Lines
P.O. Box 66045
Seattle, WA 98166

Other EMF Resources
U.S. EPA EMF Group
Office of Radiation Programs
401 M Street, S.W.
Washington, DC 20460

California Public Utilities Commission Compliance Division
505 Van Ness Avenue
Room 3102
San Francisco, CA 94102
(415) 557-4027

New York State Power Lines Project
NYS Department of Health, School of Public Health
11 University Place
Albany, NY 12203

Resources for Books on Water
Fluoride: The Aging Factor
Dr. John Yiamouyannis
Health Action Press, 1983

Water: The Element of Life
Theodor and Wolgram Schwenk, 1990
Based on the Rudolf Steiner philosophy, explores many
dimensions of water.
Anthroposophic Press
RR 4, Box 94A1
Hudson, NY 12534
(518) 851-2054
$15.95 plus $2.25 s&h

Danger on Tap: The Government's Failure to Enforce the
Federal Safe Drinking Water Act (1988)
National Wildlife Federation
1400 16th Street, N.W.
Washington, DC 20036
(202) 797-6800
Free.

Organizations
Food and Water
RR 1, Box 30
Old Schoolhouse Common
Marshfield, VT 05658
A consumer advocacy organization focusing on food and
water. Subscribe to their quarterly newsletter.

Water Testing
To test your source of drinking water (the prices are just
to give you a range; contact the companies for details):

Water Test Corp.
33 South Commercial Street
Manchester, NH 03101
(800) 426-8378/(603) 623-7400

To check for lead, copper, PCB, nitrates, radium, uranium: $250. Strontium: $75. Heavy metals: $90.

National Testing Laboratories
6151 Wilson Mills Road
Cleveland, OH 44143
(216) 449-2525/(800) 458-3330
Lead alone: $29. 14 metals, organic compounds, bacteria, 20 pesticides: $119.

Suburban Water Testing Labs
4600 Kutztown Road
Temple, PA 19560
(800) 433-6595
Lead: $19. Lead, pesticides, metals, and others: $390.

Water Research Institute
P.O. Box 930
Blue Hill, ME 04614
(207) 374-2384
They test water by a unique photographic process. They also promote a sort of waterfall called "formflow."

Klabin Marketing
(212) 877-3632
Kits to check for lead in water.

For information on chemicals in water:
Environmental Health Unit, Bureau of Health
Robert Frakes, M.D.
(207) 289-3378

Lead Information Center, National Safety Council
(800) LEAD-FYI

Keep in mind that by law you are entitled to see the results of water tests conducted on your municipal system. Contact the local water utility and ask for information on contaminants in your drinking water, by the authority of your state's health department. Call your nearest EPA office (there are eight around the country) and ask for the nearest EPA-certified lab that tests public drinking water systems.

▲

"Despite growing interest in the fate of the planet, nothing short of sharp changes will rescue the Earth's ailing eco-systems from destruction."
—*The 1992 Annual Report of the WorldWatch Institute*

▲

EPA Safe Drinking Water Hotline
(800) 426-4791
Ask for the number of your local EPA division of water quality.

EPA Regional Offices
Listed in local telephone directories.

Water Quality Association
4151 Naperville Road
Lisle, IL 60532
(708) 505-0160

Water Spoken Here
67 Denata Square
Wheaton, IL 60187

Various Products to Purify Water
Aerobic o7
Aerobic Life Products
Phoenix, AZ 85040
5–20 drops in 8 ounces of water, or for storage 20 drops
per gallon. 2 ounces, $13.

Willard Water
CAW Industries
Rapid City, SD 57702

Rio Grand Marketing
Fargo, ND 58102
2 ounces for each gallon of cleaned water.

Bottled Water
For water to be clean it must be from a deep source.
Surface water is eventually contaminated by runoff and fallout.
The deepest source in the United States is:
Mountain Valley Spring
(800) 638-2323

Clean the Air
Summertime Products
508 D Street, S.E.
Auburn, WA 98002
(206) 833-6604
Use nature's own ozone oxygen to sterilize the air you
breath with the Ozonator. Rids air of harmful
microbacteria.

To eliminate allergens from your home or office use the
indoor air purifier based on NASA-type technology. It
removes contaminants at o.3 micron size, pollens,

bacteria, room dust from a room 20' by 20'. Cost about $299.

Enviracaire portable high efficiency air cleaner
Life Service Supplements
3535 Hwy #66 Bldg 2
Neptune, NJ 07753
(800) 542-3232

Save the Trees
Global Relief
P.O. Box 2000
Department GR2
Washington, DC 20013

Reforest the Earth Project
48 Bethel Street
Norwich
Norfolk NR2 INR
England

Rainforest Action Network
301 Broadway
San Francisco, CA 94133
(415) 398-4404

Read About the State of the World
State of the World: Annual Report on the Global Environment
Lester Brown et al.
Worldwatch Institute
1776 Massachusetts Avenue
Washington, DC 20036
(202) 452-1999
$9.95 per copy, discounts on larger orders.

Understand the Interrelation of All Things
World As Lover, World As Self
Joanna Macy
Parallax Press, 1991
A collection of talks and essays on the understanding that all our world is an extension of ourselves.

Environment Information by Computer Link-up
The WELL (Whole Earth 'Lectronic Link)
(415) 332-4335
Fact sharing and consensus building over your computer. 9–5 weekdays PST or modem into (415) 332-6106 or through CompuServe node, host WELL.

Some Books for Information on the Environment
The Environmental Almanac
Compiled by the World Resources Institute
Houghton Mifflin, 1993
600 pages of facts.

The Environmental Address Book: How to Reach the Environment's Greatest Champions and Worst Offenders
Michael Levine
Perigee Books, 1991
A good listing of good leads.

Save Our Planet: 750 Everyday Ways You Can Help Clean Up the Earth
Diane MacEachern
Dell Books, 1990
Concise, clear, full of facts.

Earthright: Every Citizen's Guide
Patricia Hynes
Prima Publishing, 1990
A good resource for informed action.

Who Is Who in Service to the Earth
ed. Hans Keller
Vision Link Education Foundation, 1992
A 500-page book listing of people, projects, and
organizations who are working for a healthy Earth habitat
for humans. To order:
Vision Link
P.O. Box 448
Waynesville, NC 28786
($30, plus $2.50 postage)

The Greenpeace Guide to Anti-Environmental Organizations
Odonian Press
P.O. Box 7776
Berkeley, CA 94707
A description of groups with deliberately misleading
names who are not working for benefit of the
environment but are only green facades. ($7 including
postage)

Early Environmental Thoughts
Desert Solitaire
Edward Abbey
Simon & Schuster, 1968

A Thousand Mile Walk to the Gulf
John Muir
Penguin Books, 1992

Magazines
E
P.O. Box 6667
Syracuse, NY 13217
Send for a free trial issue. 6 issues, $20.

Buzzworm
P.O. Box 2907
Boulder, CO 80329
6 issues, $21.

Some Resources for Recordings of Sounds of the Earth and of Earth's Peoples to Inspire Its Preservation

Celestial Harmonies
P.O. Box 30122
Tucson, AZ 85751
(602) 326-4400
Music of sacred ceremonies.

Elektra Nonesuch
75 Rockefeller Plaza
New York, NY 10019
(212) 484-7200
Ethnic music.

Living Music
P.O. Box 72
Litchfield, CT 06759
(203) 567-8796
Sounds of mammals and animals.

Nature Recordings
P.O. Box 2749
Friday Harbor, WA 98250
(800) 228-5711
Sounds of nature.

Rykodisc
  Pickering Wharf, Building C
  Salem, MA 01970
  (508) 744-7678
  Sounds of nature and indigenous voices.

ABOUT THE AUTHOR

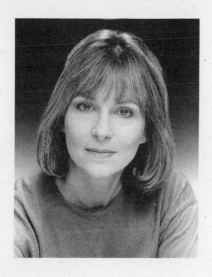

Sara Shannon is a health researcher and writer who is particularly concerned about the relationship of the health of the earth to human health, and, in turn, how human health affects judgments which determine the state of the health of the earth. Her first book, *Diet for the Atomic Age*, focused on this topic.

She lives in New York City, pending moving to a beautiful farm.